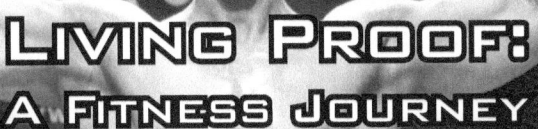

LIVING PROOF:
A FITNESS JOURNEY

BY

LEE J. ROUPAS

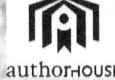

authorHOUSE®

DISCLAIMER

The author of this book is neither a dietitian nor a medical professional. All health-related matters require supervision. Please consult and obtain clearance from a physician before performing any of the exercises or following any of the suggestions in this book. The author and publisher deny any liability that may arise directly or indirectly from the use of this book.

AuthorHouse™
1663 Liberty Drive, Suite 200
Bloomington, IN 47403
www.authorhouse.com
Phone: 1-800-839-8640

First published by AuthorHouse 4/14/2009

ISBN: 978-1-4389-2582-0 (sc)

Printed in the United States of America
Bloomington, Indiana

This book is printed on acid-free paper.

In loving memory of my grandparents,
the most influential people in my life:

Leo and Ann Roupas

Gus "Remo" and Estelle Kopan

AUTHOR'S NOTE

This book is for the hard gainers; for those who are too intimidated to step into a gym; for those confused or duped by the gimmicks in the fitness industry; for the ones who get ridiculed for being too skinny or too fat; for the athletes who did not make the team because they were not big or strong enough. I commend the ones who do it naturally.

ACKNOWLEDGMENTS AND SPECIAL THANKS

A successful journey in life is not made alone, but with the support, guidance, and a little help from friends. I want to acknowledge some of the people who have assisted and supported me in writing this book. I also want to express my gratitude to people whom I have encountered in my journey in life who have impacted or changed my life to bring me where I am today.

Ken Muellner—a good friend who has stood by me, and who gave me the bug to write this book.

Chuck Sanow—the owner of USA Gym: a friend, a mentor, and a classy individual for many years.

Dr. John Stavrakos—a lifelong loyal friend, John has stood with me during the darkest times of my life.

Paul Baltz—a man who is brutally honest, who I call the "Michael Jordan" of writing and proofreading. He has been a big help in this project.

Bob Albertini—a man who has assisted me nutritionally, and whose knowledge has contributed to some of the principles in this fitness/ bodybuilding book that have benefited me and others over the years.

Lex Luger—a man whose friendship and great example of fitness have guided a significant part of my fitness journey.

Juan "Mr. Karate" Hernandez—a friend who has been like an older brother to me, and whose toughness and honesty have kept me on a straight path.

George Bliss—a dear friend and my publicist.

I also would like to express my utmost gratitude to a highly talented photographer, *Rick Drew,* who did a phenomenal job with the photographs. And I would like to give my heartfelt appreciation to the models how helped make this fitness book possible:

Jeremy Coleman—a former Marine who competed in his first bodybuilding competition under my guidance and won his weight class. He has a big career ahead in the sport. Like me, Jeremy is doing it naturally.

Anna Chronos—a certified Pilates instructor, model, and my cousin. You can tell Anna stays in great shape.

Kelly Kearney—a figure competitor who entered her first competition in 2007 at age 19. Kelly trains hard, and I commend her for stepping up at a young age.

Finally, special thanks go to my parents, *John and Kathy Roupas*; my brother, *Dean,* and his lovely wife, *Laura*; and my sister, *Stacie,* for their love and support throughout the years.

CONTENTS

Preface: Seven Reasons to Read This Book   xiii

Introduction   1

Chapter 1: The Skinny Kid Who Started the Journey   5

Chapter 2: The Opposite End of the Spectrum   15

Chapter 3: Before Beginning a Fitness Journey   19

Chapter 4: Guidance for the Journey   23

Chapter 5: Program Design Suggestions for Everyone   35

Chapter 6: Warming Up, Cooling Down, and Stretching   51

Chapter 7: Body Parts, Targeted Muscles,
            and Exercises for Building a Nice Physique   63
            Chest   64
            Shoulders   68
            Back   72
            Biceps   78
            Triceps   82
            Legs   88
            Abdominals   94

Chapter 8: Core Training and Ball Exercises   101

Chapter 9: Continuing the Journey and Moving Forward   123

PREFACE:
SEVEN REASONS TO READ THIS BOOK

"Every journey begins with the first step." This often-repeated adage may be something of a cliché, but it's still true—especially when the journey is about improving your health and fitness.

Life itself is a journey. When embarking on one of life's journeys, the first step is to have a vision, a goal, and a plan. No matter what area of life you want to improve—professional, financial, physical—you need discipline. Without discipline, you will fail in life. That's a strong statement, I know, but it's meant to be a reality check. I want to assure you that I am speaking also about myself with this statement. I, too, need to reinforce the principle and good lifestyle habit of discipline.

Discipline is required for a healthy, productive life. It also can mean the difference between a purposeful and fulfilling life, and a life of regrets. Without structure and proper discipline, life is filled with clutter and disorganization. A professor once gave me this definition: "Discipline is doing what needs to be done, when it should be done, and in the manner in which it should be done, regardless of how a person feels or what a person wants to do." Discipline takes sacrifice. The champion athlete is the athlete who does what the other competitors will not do, or are not willing to do, to win. If it means spending more time training and perfecting skills, strengthening every weakness, the achiever will sacrifice pleasure to win.

Health and fitness is a lifelong journey that requires discipline. As a fitness professional, I encounter people who blatantly admit they do not have the discipline to work out. Unfortunately, it be may be too late for some people who neglect their health. There are individuals who go a whole lifetime without exercising, with improper nutrition, living stressful lives that eventually catch up with them in the form of illness. A fitness journey is a pursuit of healthy, functional living. Though not pleasant at times because of the effort required, the benefits of good health are priceless and long term.

I am writing this book to encourage you to start a journey toward fitness. If you already work out consistently, or if you've been training for several years, my hope is that this book will help you to take your physique, conditioning, and health to the next level.

In this book, I share my own journey. I discuss circumstances I have faced and obstacles that I've met along the way. My journey has covered twenty-five years of my life. It began the first time I picked up a weight, and continued through my years as a collegiate and amateur athlete to my arrival as a champion, competitive, drug-free bodybuilder. "Drug-free" means that throughout my fitness journey and athletic career, I have not taken any anabolic steroids, human growth hormone, or any other performance-enhancing drugs.

In this book, I share exercise routines and workout techniques I have used during more than twenty-five years of serious training to develop my physique. Because of my persistence—my discipline—in doing these exercises, I have been able to compete as a drug-free bodybuilder, and to live a healthy life.

When I walk into any bookstore, I find a solid wall of fitness books. When I skim some, I find a lack of clarity. What makes this book different is that it is written for people at all levels of fitness, athleticism, and bodybuilding. This is the unique story of a "regular guy" from Chicago who went from being skinny to being an overweight participant in athletics to becoming a champion, natural bodybuilder.

This book has something for everyone. The novice can get a good start; regular workout veterans can explore new techniques to add new twists to their workout programs; and bodybuilders preparing for their first contests can find tips and guidance.

This book is for *you!* The tools and knowledge are here.

Writing this book has been a journey in and of itself. A lot of this book has been written while traveling between cities in my busy schedule. I wrote this book in hotels, airports, and even on the commuter train to my job in downtown Chicago. In putting this book together, I did a lot of research, I explored new exercise techniques, and I pulled together twenty-five years' worth of "old school" techniques that still work and will always work.

Here, then, are seven reasons to read this book:

1. To gain an understanding of the value of fitness.
2. To set goals not only in fitness, but in other areas of life—regardless of age.
3. To learn from and be inspired by a person who did it the old-fashioned way, without "gimmicks" or performance-enhancing drugs.
4. To develop the discipline and motivation necessary to make working out an everyday lifestyle habit.
5. To learn proper stretching and exercise techniques so as to prevent injury, build lean muscle, and improve cardiovascular health.
6. To know which exercises to perform for each body part.
7. To experience the benefits of fitness for functional living.

This is a book you can take with you to the gym. It is intended to educate, motivate, and invigorate you with the tools to achieve your fitness goals. The contents, fitness principles, and exercises are easy to apply.

Now, let's embark on a journey!

—*Lee Roupas*

INTRODUCTION

When I started weight training in the 1980s, I spent a significant amount of time reading bodybuilding magazines. When I went to the grocery store with my mother, I went to the magazine section and pulled out the bodybuilding and fitness magazines to read while my mother shopped. The magazines sparked my curiosity and inspired me to want to look like the musclemen in the magazines. I read the exercise tips offered by some of the featured bodybuilders in the magazines. It was my way of researching, and I would try to persuade my mother to buy me the magazine so I could try some of the weight-training techniques.

In our old house, my dad had a few weights lying around, and I tried to lift them. I used the weights to try the exercises I saw in the magazines.

In 1982, my dad bought my brother and me a weight set and a bench. This was one of the best gifts a father could give his sons. I put this weight set and bench to good use while I experimented with different magazine tips in high hopes of building muscle. From that day in 1982 to the present, lifting weights has been a big part of my life.

The years of grueling training were put to the test when I entered my first bodybuilding contest. It was a typical cold, crisp, bone-chilling Chicago winter day, but I didn't feel it. My focus was on the task ahead. I was in the best shape of my life, and very confident about my look. My body fat that morning must have been around three percent. I couldn't drink any water, and the only thing that kept my energy level up was my adrenaline. Nothing mattered to me but to get to the competition and hold my mandatory poses on stage, in front of the judges and the other competitors, with every ounce of my being.

It was an hour's drive west from Chicago to a big auditorium in Elgin, Illinois. The ride seemed longer because I was "carb-depleted"— low on both carbohydrates and energy.

When I arrived at the auditorium, I saw that I blended in with this unique group of athletes. This elite group makes up a very small segment of the population. They stand out everywhere they go. They can easily be spotted in a shopping mall, grocery store, or restaurant. They are stared at, and are sometimes admonished with rude comments by insecure people. They also sometimes receive admiration from those who appreciate hard work, dedication, and discipline. The type of people I am talking about are bodybuilders, and I had finally become one of them.

Wherever I go, I am noticed. I am six feet three inches tall, and I weigh 245 to 250 pounds in my off-season when I'm not dieting for a bodybuilding contest. I'm aware of the stares when I walk into a room. Sometimes people ask me to flex. One night at a Chicago nightclub, a gentleman complimented my physique and challenged me to arm wrestle. I thanked him for his kind words, but I replied, "You are probably a ringer" (a slang term for a person who does not appear to be good at a skill, but in reality is very good). Another time, I was walking my dog at a strip mall in my neighborhood when an older gentleman yelled out his car window, "Hey, young man, want to arm wrestle?"

Who would have thought so many years ago that Lee, the skinny kid who rode his bike and ran around the neighborhood, would one day be stepping on a bodybuilding stage? My body was oiled up and dowsed with tanning spray, and my muscle tone was nicely defined. It was time to display my best shape to a panel of judges and a crowd in the big auditorium. I flexed and held each mandatory pose to the point of pure exhaustion.

I had spent twenty months preparing for my first bodybuilding contest. I trained five to six days a week, performing grueling workouts and pushing my body beyond endurance. It meant strict discipline and sacrifice, with countless hours spent training, dieting, and practicing my posing. The contest preparation also included time spent tanning, preparing my meals, and finding time to rest.

It came down to nine mandatory poses that lasted no more than five minutes. The contest preparation was a small journey. A journey like no other—and one that turned out to be a time of glory when I won my weight class.

It was a goal set and a goal accomplished.

CHAPTER 1:
THE SKINNY KID WHO
STARTED THE JOURNEY

While I was growing up in the 1970s, bodybuilding was beginning to gain popularity. Prominent bodybuilders such as Lou Ferrigno, Arnold Schwarzenegger, and Franco Colombo helped put the sport of bodybuilding into the media spotlight. I admired these athletes when I saw them on television or in magazines, and I especially enjoyed watching Ferrigno's starring role on TV's *The Incredible Hulk*. I was in awe of Ferrigno's physique, given his height of six feet five inches.

I was a skinny kid, and I hated it. I was ridiculed by friends and relatives. My friend from my old neighborhood, Sam Di Franco, often reminded me how skinny I was when he saw me walking down the street. But no matter how much I ate, I could not gain any weight. As a preteen I participated in a local age-grouped swim team, but my skinny build made me feel uncomfortable around the other swimmers.

I was fortunate to have a father who made physical fitness and participation in athletics a high priority in his life, and encouraged me to do the same. My dad began lifting weights in the 1970s. After work, he trained at a gym; at home, he talked about his training with enthusiasm. When he bought my brother and me our first weight set, he took the time to demonstrate exercises for each body part. I was excited at the thought of gaining some muscle size, so I did the exercises on my own. My favorite exercise was doing single bicep curls over the edge of the couch. I wanted my skinny arms to look like the arms I admired in the magazines.

I was doing well at my swim meets, and my dad wanted to help me improve my performance. In the mid-1980s, he was kind enough to buy me a membership at his health club. I wanted to increase muscle size and gain more strength to better pull myself through the water.

My dad worked out religiously at the gym. It was there that he met John Hansen, a well-known bodybuilding champion in the Chicago area. John taught my dad some exercises and put him on a workout program. My dad then taught me how to follow the program. I saw my dad making some gains and looking better, and that sparked my enthusiasm even more.

In my junior year of high school, I started weight training with my father after school. The gym was conveniently located across the street from my high school.

The first time I walked into the gym, I saw some big men lifting heavy weights. I heard all the grunts and groans as the men lifted and then slammed the weights back on the rack. There was loud music blasting, and the place was full of sweat and energy. As an athlete, I felt energized. I was inspired by the intensity that the men in the gym showed in lifting heavy weights. My dad knew everyone and introduced me to the members. The atmosphere was positive and encouraging. Everyone was supportive of one another, and I enjoyed the sense of camaraderie.

The first time I trained with my dad, we worked on our chest muscles. This was the start of a new season in my fitness journey. I began by using light weights to help me learn the form and technique, and to understand which muscles were being worked for growth and development.

Learning the correct form and proper exercise technique is the first step in muscle growth, body change, and injury prevention. It remains a top priority for my individual workouts as a bodybuilder today. As a certified fitness trainer, I stress the importance of proper lifting technique to my clients. That's a big factor in my "injury-free" record among my clients: no client of mine has been injured under my watch, and I plan to keep that streak going. In the gym, however, I often see that form is compromised for heavy lifting. There is no room for ego while training in the gym if you want to train correctly and remain injury-free. Proper form helps you to fully work the muscle group and muscle fibers for growth.

For two months, my father and I trained consistently. I began to see pleasing results. My body began to change as muscle was added to my 160-pound frame. My strength increased, and I felt more energetic.

When the swim season began again in late fall, I continued to weight train, and I saw a difference in my performance. I was a stronger swimmer, and my swim times kept improving. I weight trained all through my senior year in high school, but I stopped when the swim season was over and I graduated.

After graduation, I worked a summer job in a warehouse to make money for college. I was planning to attend Michigan State University in the fall of 1988. The job in the warehouse required heavy lifting. Though I was no longer going to the gym, lifting heavy boxes and drums kept me in good-enough shape to maintain muscular definition and lean body mass.

The summer of 1988 is on record as one of the hottest summers in Chicago. Temperatures ranged from 90 to 100 degrees for days—outside *and* inside the warehouse. The constant heat, sweating, and moving around all helped me keep my lean physique.

When I arrived at the Michigan State University campus, working out was not on my mind. Instead, I drank, partied, and stayed out late on the weekends, wreaking havoc on my physique. One night, toward the end of the winter quarter of my freshman year, I took off my shirt in my dorm room and looked in the mirror. I was very displeased with what I saw. By the time I came home for my winter break, I had already gained the often-talked-about "freshman fifteen." The freshman fifteen is the amount of weight incoming freshmen often gain from the time they enter college to the time they come home for winter break. The factors responsible for my freshman fifteen were living a sedentary lifestyle, overeating, and drinking alcohol. (Here I was, away from home and drinking underage. Today I am a spokesperson against underage drinking. I share those experiences when I travel the country speaking to young people.)

The stress of my college courses also contributed to my unplanned weight gain. The muscle tone I once had was gone, and I had more body fat than usual. This was a wake-up call for me to start taking care of my body again. It was time for me to quit drinking alcohol, clean up my eating, and start training in the gym.

The summer after my freshman year of college, I got a job working for a long-time family friend who had a milk-delivery business. I worked on a truck, delivering milk and dairy products to restaurants all over the Chicago area. Like my summer job from the previous year, this job also required a lot of lifting. Not only was it hard manual labor, but the workday was long: my boss and I worked fourteen-hour days, on average. Despite the long workday I still found time to train at a gym.

The long days and constant moving from delivery stop to delivery stop also increased my appetite. I ate at several restaurants where we delivered products. With all the working out and eating out that I did, my body weight increased from 170 pounds at the start of my freshman year to 185 pounds that summer.

When I returned for my second year at Michigan State University, I received compliments from friends who noticed I had gotten bigger. This is what I wanted to hear, and it meant my efforts had paid off. The compliments also were a good incentive to continue training and build more muscle mass. Training also helped me get through my classes. I had had problems in the past concentrating on my studies, but I found that working out improved my concentration.

I established a daily routine: after I finished my classes each day, I went back to the dorm and rested to muster the energy for my workouts. When I finished my workouts, I returned again to the dorm, showered, and went to the cafeteria to supply my body with the proper nutrients for muscle growth. (Of course, during my college years, I didn't have the nutritional knowledge that I have today. As I look back, I see that I did not always eat properly, but that, too, became part of my fitness journey; I learned as I progressed.) After I finished eating, I would gather my books, notes, and backpack, and go study at the library. I couldn't get anything done in my dorm room—there were too many distractions and too many people dropping in on me.

Throughout my college years, training remained a part of my daily routine, just like brushing my teeth. I made substantial gains in muscle mass during my junior year, and I continued to train consistently when I went home for the summer. In June 1992, the summer before my last year at Michigan State, I enrolled in martial arts training to develop my mental discipline and focus, and to improve my fighting skills. The years I spent in martial arts training proved helpful to me later when I worked as a "doorman"—a polite term for a bouncer at nightclubs and other events. There were times I had to defend myself or get a rowdy patron into a submission hold. My martial arts training also played a crucial role in my individual fitness journey. I couldn't have chosen a better form of conditioning: martial arts built up my cardiovascular system and increased my muscle strength and endurance.

It was vital for me to enter my senior year at Michigan State in top physical condition because I had made the cheerleading squad. Cheerleading is one sport where strength and conditioning are of utmost importance. The sport required me to be able to lift a partner for stunts, and to have the endurance to last for four quarters of a football game. When Spartan Stadium was filled to capacity, our squad had to help a crowd of more than 74,000 fans follow the game enthusiastically.

On the days that I didn't have cheerleading practice, I continued to follow the routine and workout program that I had developed during my sophomore year, which kept me in shape for my sport. I received compliments on my physique from fellow students, fans, and alumni, some of whom said that I should be out playing on the football team. Compliments can really motivate a person to continue to train and to set new goals, and they certainly did that for me.

I graduated from Michigan State in 1993 and returned home to Chicago, where I immediately joined a local health club. I also did more research, read more books, and learned more about bodybuilding. I continued my usual workout activities: weight training and martial arts. Now that I was working in the professional world, I experienced different stresses and circumstances than I had as a college student, and my way to relieve stress was to work out. Unfortunately, people who don't have a way to deal with stress may find that it damages their health.

In the spring of 1995, my brother found a gym that he decided to join. When I saw him after a workout at his new gym, he couldn't stop talking about it. My membership at the health club was nearing expiration, and I had been thinking about making a change. I decided to visit his gym and see if it was a place at which I would like to train. When I drove up to the parking lot, I saw a big sign on the building: "USA GYM." As soon as I walked in, I liked the atmosphere. It was a "hardcore gym"—a place for people who work out seriously and still use old but durable equipment. USA Gym is one of the few remaining hardcore gyms in Chicago. A lot of the hardcore and independently owned gyms have gone out of business due to the emergence of corporate gyms, but USA Gym has stood for twenty-two years against the big franchises.

And so I began another chapter of my fitness journey by joining USA Gym. I was inspired not only by the atmosphere, but also by the intensity and hard work of the members. Their enthusiasm gave me the incentive to train harder and gain more muscle size. I had one problem, though: I was a "hard gainer." Hard gainers are people who have difficulty gaining muscle mass. No matter how often hard gainers may train, or how heavy the weights they use, they do not see a change in their physiques.

Recognizing that I was a hard gainer, I stepped back and analyzed what I was doing. I realized that I was overtraining—training too much and too often, and not giving my body the rest necessary for muscle and cellular recovery. In addition, I was still doing martial arts training, because I was working security at nightclubs and other events. While the weight training helped make my strikes and kicks more powerful, the martial arts training made it even more difficult for me to gain muscle.

In 1999, an injury brought my martial arts career to an end. I was going for a promotion test for my next belt, and I had to spar with a fellow student. He and I took the match to the ground as we attempted to get one another in a submission hold. The dojo, or training hall, had an old wooden floor. After I put a submission hold on the other student, I looked down and saw a big gash at the top of my right shinbone. I could not feel any pain at the time, because my mind was so focused and my adrenaline was working. Any pain anywhere in my body had been blocked out of my mind. In fact, part of the test involved blocking out pain. We had to stand still while Sensei Bob Lee took a stick and struck us hard across the chest. We could not flinch. When one of the three students being tested did flinch, Sensei Lee kept hitting him with the stick until he was able to take the hit standing still.

When the two-day test ended, I felt like I had just returned from fighting a war or boxing Mike Tyson. I went home, noticed the big welt across my chest, and cleaned the sizeable gash on my leg. Three days later, my sister noticed that my leg was infected. I had a little pain in the infected area, but I hadn't paid attention to it; I was trained to block out pain and endure injuries. I was stubborn and bullheaded, and I didn't want to go to the emergency room. After much nagging from my sister, I finally got in the car. At the emergency room, it was determined that not only was my leg infected, the infection was spreading. The doctor immediately started me on antibiotics. I spent a week in the hospital, and had to take five weeks off work. I had an intravenous (IV) line in my arm through which antibiotics were administered every eight hours. I lost twenty-five pounds—most of it muscle mass that I had worked so hard to gain. I could not lift weights or do any strenuous activity. If my sister hadn't gotten me to the hospital, my leg would have had to be amputated, or I might even have died. It was enough to put the fear of God in me. After I recovered and got the approval of the doctor, I returned to the gym.

In July 1999, I met Bob Albertini, a nutritionist who also trained at USA Gym. Bob and I connected. We had a lot in common: we were both bodybuilders, both black belts, and we both had Mediterranean backgrounds—mine Greek, his Italian. He used to work security at nightclubs, as I did, and we liked similar qualities in a woman. Under Bob's expert guidance, I was able to restore my health through proper diet, supplementation, and lifestyle adjustments. He was instrumental in helping me to improve my physique and maintain my good health.

Once I was fully recovered, I was able to resume my normal life and intensify my training. Within two months, I had gained back the twenty-five pounds I had lost. In the gym world, regaining muscle after taking time off from training is called "muscle memory." Thank God for muscle memory!

During the time that I was off, I reevaluated my life. I felt the urge to retire from martial arts and embark on a new chapter in my fitness journey: bodybuilding. I made the decision to do bodybuilding naturally, without anabolic steroids or growth hormone. It was now time to accomplish a goal I had set in my junior year at Michigan State University in 1991: I wanted to compete in a bodybuilding competition. I had already accomplished my goals in martial arts; now I felt that it was time to work toward a new goal.

In 2000, I started training with USA Gym owner and International Federation of Bodybuilding (IFBB) professional bodybuilder Chuck Sanow. Chuck holds more than twenty bodybuilding titles, and he has trained several champions. He earned his professional bodybuilding card when he was in his mid-forties after several years of near-misses. He's an example of why age should not deter anyone from accomplishing a goal. He is one of the hardest workers I know, both professionally and as a bodybuilder. After I saw how he helped other competitors, I knew I could trust Chuck's expertise in bodybuilding contest preparation.

Training with Chuck has refined my physique. His workouts can be grueling, especially on the days that we train legs. Chuck often jokes, "I like to see a grown man cry." One Saturday afternoon after a leg workout with Chuck, I threw up in the parking lot. On another occasion, I passed out in the locker room after a strenuous leg workout.

At the beginning of 2001, I asked Chuck if I was ready to compete. He nodded his head with approval. I was thrilled that I was about to achieve a goal I had set ten years earlier. Chuck gave me a diet to follow for my contest preparation. He also demonstrated the eight mandatory poses on which competitors are judged. Once I learned the mandatory poses, it was time to put together my one-minute posing routine.

For twelve weeks I was under Chuck's guidance, and I carefully followed his instructions. My life was work, train, and sleep. During the off-season, when I was building my physique but not dieting, I weighed 230 pounds. By following Chuck's diet, I weighed 197 pounds by the morning of the competition. I found that if you listen to your coaches, teachers, or mentors, you can achieve success. As a result, I won my weight class in the Illinois Natural Novice Championships.

I did not enter my first contest expecting to win. I stepped on the bodybuilding stage to have fun and to show off the best physical condition of my life. But the victory made all the sacrifices, including curtailing my social life, well worth it. The dieting, the hours spent training in the gym, the strict discipline: it was all worth it to achieve my goal.

Is this something I would do again? Absolutely! This first contest ignited a desire in me to keep competing. Bodybuilders, as well as average people working out in the gym, should challenge themselves to improve their physical bodies yearly.

Lastly, if a 150-pound skinny kid with normal ability can do it, you certainly can!

CHAPTER 2:
THE OPPOSITE END
OF THE SPECTRUM

I am sharing my personal fitness journey with you in this book. So far I have been candid about obstacles I encountered along my journey. I want to show you, the reader, that I am an average human being. I am not one of those models you see on television or in the magazines. I am a person with a desire to get fit and stay healthy. As both a "regular" person and a fitness professional, I do not suggest gimmicks or get-fit-quick schemes. I want to show you that I did it through hard work and proper technique—and you can, too. As I mentioned in the previous chapter, I did not have a good physique at the start of my journey. It is my hope that I clearly demonstrate in this book how you can achieve this look using the techniques and principles that I share here.

As age creeps up, it becomes more difficult to lose pounds and maintain a healthy weight. Therefore, hard, consistent work must be done to keep body fat at a healthy level. After my first contest in 2001, I acquired a competitive fervor. I competed in three more bodybuilding contests because it was enjoyable. When my competition season ended in 2002, I attained an off-season weight of 240 pounds—ten pounds higher than in the previous year. Later in 2003, some changes in my professional and personal life put more stress on my mind, body, and soul. My job starting getting hectic; I was traveling and working long hours. Between working my day job and training clients in the evening,

I was busy an average of twelve to fourteen hours a day. When I was traveling, I found myself consuming large amounts of junk food from gas stations to stay awake while I was driving. The long hours and traveling exhausted me to the point that I could not train consistently. It was not long before I did what I did in my freshman year in college: I looked in the mirror. I had more body fat than I normally do. When I got on the scale, I weighed 252 pounds. My muscle definition was nonexistent. My appearance and my lack of energy were caused by stress, bad eating, and too many missed workouts.

In early 2004, I did a photo shoot and took some headshots. When my photographer showed me the photos, I noticed weight gain in my face. When I put on my suits, the jackets were tight and the pants did not fit in the waistline. I felt sluggish, and I was disappointed at what I had allowed to happen to my body. The stress, unhealthy eating, and inconsistent workouts also negatively influenced my mental state.

That time in my life was a nightmare. I was not being the "living proof" or a good example of a fitness trainer. I knew it was time to get back to a consistent workout routine, eliminate this excess weight, and regain mental balance.

The upside of this experience: I found myself on the opposite end of the spectrum. Eighteen short months ago, I had won a bodybuilding title. Now it was time to make a comeback, and that's why I titled this book *Living Proof: A Fitness Journey*, because it is a journey. All I can say is: I've been there! Don't be discouraged—it happens. But something *can* be done. I took immediate steps, and I had the determination to change my body.

Around this same time, I agreed to do a modeling job scheduled for later in the year. I also was asked to participate in a celebrity golf outing, being a well-known media personality in the Chicago area. I'd be signing autographs at the golf outing to raise money for Alicia's House, a food pantry that feeds and makes holidays possible for hundreds of families. It was founded by my friend, Juan "Mr. Karate" Hernandez, in honor of his granddaughter Alicia, who passed away at age four and who had a heart for people. I was honored to volunteer and be part of this event every year.

I had five months to get in shape for the modeling job and the golf outing, because they were both the same weekend.

It was time to put all my knowledge—everything I'm sharing in this book—to practice. The new short-term goal was to get in good shape for the events to come. I trained diligently and consistently, and my body started to look the way it should. It took me three months to go from a weight of 252 pounds—the heaviest I have been—to 240 pounds. Once back to my 240-pound, off-season shape, I even started seeing some abdominals.

Once I had dropped the twelve pounds of body fat and improved my appearance, I felt the urge to compete again in bodybuilding. It had now been three years since I had competed in a contest; injuries as well as work-related travel had kept me on the sidelines. But now I put my mind into competitive mode, called Chuck Sanow, and started preparing for the next contest. I was still busy with work, travel, and training clients, even in the midst of my contest preparation. The challenge was—and is—to balance every area of my life.

The contest was scheduled for November 2005. My life consisted of eating, sleeping, working, and training. I also had enrolled in graduate school that fall, so I had to find time to study, too. My social life became extinct.

The morning of the contest, I was in my best condition. Through rigorous diet and training, my weight had now dropped to 201 pounds. My body was ripped and hard.

I left my house at 6:30 AM for breakfast. Chuck had given me strict orders regarding what to eat in the morning. The contest was in Belvidere, Illinois, about two hours north of Chicago near Rockford, Illinois. While I was driving, I popped in my tape of Journey, a famous 1980s rock band. I turned up the volume, and their ever-popular song, "Don't Stop Believing," played loudly in the car. It was the theme song of the 2005 Chicago White Sox, who two weeks earlier had won the World Series. I was jubilant, being a lifelong, diehard Chicago White

Sox fan from the south side of Chicago. Watching the Sox win the playoffs and World Series had encouraged me while I was training. The team's tenacity capped by their victory was inspirational. Now it was time for a victory of my own.

The prejudging was that morning, during which the competitors do eight mandatory poses and are compared to each other by the judges. When the head judge called out the poses, I held each pose as tightly as I could. During the second part of the contest—the evening show—the bodybuilders perform their 60-second posing routines to music. This is the fun part of competing, where I get to be a showman and perform in front of the crowd. I was the last competitor in my weight class to perform. Then the emcee called all the competitors back on stage for the awards. I had no idea where I would place, because I was competing against good physiques. To my surprise, they announced the competitor next to me as the second-place finisher, and then announced my name as the winner. When I was handed the first-place trophy, I raised my arm in victory and gave a front bicep pose. I was elated because of the sacrifice and hard work it took to prepare for this contest. This was a sweet victory after a three-year layoff. I could not have asked for a better comeback.

Since then I have competed in three more contests, and I hope to continue competing for as long as possible. I took the third-place trophy in my last three contests. My goal for each contest is to look better than I did the last time I competed. I feel bodybuilding is one of the most self-sacrificing and challenging sports, but also one of the most fun. I'm not only competing against the other bodies on stage, but also against myself. The satisfaction comes from improving my appearance each time I step on a stage. The contest prep includes maintaining a strict diet, eating every three hours, and constantly training to tweak my appearance.

Currently, I maintain a good off-season weight, eat clean, and train consistently throughout the year. My fitness journey is a way of life. Being on the "opposite end of the spectrum" with too much body fat was more than enough motivation to get me back on track. Quite frankly, that time in my life scared the devil out of me!

CHAPTER 3:
BEFORE BEGINNING A FITNESS JOURNEY

The first step in any journey: set goals. Goals help give you clear vision and purpose in your journey. Your fitness goals, just like any other goals, should be specific and measurable. Generic goals, such as "I just want to lose weight," should be avoided. Instead, your goal might be, "I want to lose weight so I can look and feel better."

When I set my goals at the beginning of each year, I make them specific. I write my goals in my journal, and I also write down the activities and steps I need to take in my life to reach those goals. For example, after my last bodybuilding contest, I wrote that my goal was to get my arms bigger so that they would be in proportion to the rest of my upper body. Underneath that, I wrote: "train arms twice a week; do exercises that will build the base of the arm; then do exercises that will build the peak of the bicep."

When setting your fitness goals, your main objective is to strive for healthy, functional living. This means that you should not get out of breath when you walk up a flight of stairs. You should be able to move objects, pick up young kids, and carry your groceries without too much strain. You should be able to cut the grass and do yard work without fatigue or injury. Your only doctor visit should be your annual physical. Of course, if you don't take care of your body and work out, later on in life you'll get to know your doctor quite well, and your hard-earned money will go toward medical bills.

Your fitness goals will depend on what you want your body to look like and how you want to feel. Most people want to feel vibrant and energetic. Injuries and family health history should be taken into consideration when setting fitness goals. For example, if your family has a history of heart disease, your goal might be to build good cardiovascular endurance.

So what are your personal fitness goals? And do you have the willingness, dedication, and focus to achieve your goals?

As a fitness trainer, I've heard all the workout excuses and roadblocks that people can come up with. But you need to realize that if you do not take care of your body, the consequences are a future of health problems. I have seen the consequences when people neglect their health. Yes, working out can seem daunting. I understand that there might be other things you'd rather do with your time. But what happens if you neglect brushing your teeth every day?

The most common excuse is the "I-don't-have-enough-time" excuse. Yes, we all have to work. Some of us have families; some have kids; some have houses to maintain; some have pets; and so on. The bottom line is this: you have to make time for *you!* I understand that if you are a parent, your children are your priority. It is the parents' duty to put their children's needs ahead of their own. However, Mom and Dad have to take care of themselves so that they can take care of their children. In the long run, children and parents can both enjoy a better quality of life.

I know a mother of two children who also is a wife and a full-time employee. She made the decision to work out early in the morning, before the rest of her family gets up. She gets her workout out of the way so that she can tend to her family. It is a decision she made because she also decided that she wanted to have enough energy to raise her children, and she wanted to look good for her husband. Now she's also a good role model to her children by showing them how physical fitness leads to good quality of life. Of course, your workout time should be scheduled for the time of day when you work out at your best (for me, that's during my lunch hour), or when it is most convenient. It all depends on your individual preference.

Before you invest time and money in a gym membership or a personal trainer, take an inventory of your life. Consider your lifestyle patterns and habits, your current health status, and your family history. Be honest with yourself and ask yourself the tough questions such as these:

- Is heart disease prevalent in your family?
- Did your grandparents or parents struggle with diabetes or any other ailments?
- Is there too much stress in your life?
- Are you engaging in behaviors that can be harmful to you?
- What are your eating habits?
- Are you taking any medications?
- Do you have any recurring injuries?

If you're working with a fitness professional, these are the kinds of questions you can expect to be asked. You must answer honestly. If you don't, your trainer can't design your program to solve your personal health and fitness issues.

Every New Year, many people make resolutions. One of the most common resolutions always is: "get into shape." Suddenly, gym and fitness-center parking lots are filled to capacity, and those who work out regularly now have to share the equipment with many more people. By the end of February, however, the fitness buzz starts dying down. As a fitness trainer, the biggest challenge is to keep the beginner interested in working out. Statistics show that 50 percent of all personal training clients around the United States will drop out within the first six months.

We live in a society that wants a "quick fix" or a magic pill. Unfortunately, the scam artists in the industry would like to make people believe that they can get into shape in a short amount of time and with little effort. The infomercials appeal to people's fears; they fall prey to the deception and buy the product, which does not produce the desired outcome. Most people don't know that much about fitness or the fitness industry. This book can equip you with the knowledge necessary to have a successful fitness journey. The gimmicks on television or in slick advertising will not get anyone into shape. It has to be done the old-fashioned way. I stick with the basic philosophy that has worked in my life and in the lives of so many others: good old-fashioned weight training, cardiovascular training, and good nutrition. It takes patience and time. The key to results is this: *be consistent and stick with the program.*

I want this book to be not only an educational tool for you, but also a means for motivation. I want to give you the good news that no matter what your age, it is never too late. Whether you're just starting out for the first time, or you're resuming your workout out after a layoff, you need to begin with the right mindset. If you have to make some lifestyle changes, make them! It all begins with the willingness to take a personal inventory of your life. Think about how much time you are willing to invest to fit workouts into your schedule. Consider how much time you spend watching television, talking on the phone, or surfing the Internet. Take some of that time and spend it on the gym, or on doing some activity in your home. Making better use of your time can help you lose the excuse that you don't have enough time to work out.

It's also important to take an inventory of your eating and sleeping. What empty calories are you allowing in your body? Are you getting proper rest? If you are eating too many carbohydrates and sugars, or you're not getting proper rest, now is the time to *stop!* Start now to break old, unhealthy habits, and diligently make good habits.

Throughout my years as a certified fitness professional, I have seen and trained many people who made lifestyle changes. By actively making changes, they improved their levels of fitness. When they improved their fitness levels, they also enhanced the quality of their lives.

I once trained a seventy-five-year-old woman who lived in a downtown Chicago high-rise overlooking Lake Michigan. This woman was a fine example of good health at her age. She trained consistently, even on the days I was not training her. This woman had more energy than women forty years younger. And she looked twenty years younger than her age. *It can be done! You can do it!*

CHAPTER 4:
GUIDANCE FOR THE JOURNEY

When I started training at the gym as a teenager, I was blessed to have someone who gave me direction and proper instruction, and who designed a program for me. Throughout my fitness journey, the right fitness experts, coaches, and martial arts instructors were in my life to give me the guidance I needed. I was shown step-by-step what to do. It also took some self-discovery on my part. By doing the exercises and trying the different machines in the gym, I was able to discover more exercises for each body part. I took the knowledge that I was taught and applied it when I trained on my own, and when I went back to the gym in college.

To get the most from your workout, you need direction and proper instruction. My main role as a fitness professional is to give my clients direction. First, I consult with them about healthy lifestyle habits; I get them "dialed in" to fitness. Then, when I'm in the gym with a client, I give the client a series of exercises to perform for the body parts we are working on that day. But before my client does anything, I get on the machine or take the dumbbell and I demonstrate proper technique; I also show which muscle we are working.

I often see people who are training hard, but who clearly don't have a clue what they are doing or how to train properly. In the gym, improper exercise technique is noticeable. I also notice people who perform the same routine over and over, but who don't give their muscles the proper "shock" they need to grow and develop. I might see the same people week after week, year after year, who have no changes in their physiques because they just perform the same routines repetitively. Sometimes I'd like to help them out, but I'm a person who minds his own business. Advice is not always welcomed in the gym. The gym staff should take notice and offer gentle counsel if they observe a gym member doing something that could possibly result in injury.

Your workout should be designed to meet your fitness goals. Training should be geared specifically toward weight loss, muscle toning, sculpting, bodybuilding, improving cardiovascular endurance, or whatever your individual goal is. Workouts also can be designed to enhance an athlete's performance in a particular sport. Workout programs should take into account the type of exercise, order of the exercise, number of sets, number of repetitions, rest periods, and intensity.

I strongly suggest hiring a certified personal trainer. Great athletes all have a coach or mentor in their lives. Michael Jordan, one of or the greatest players who ever stepped onto a basketball court, had a coach. A certified personal trainer can show you how to employ proper techniques to perform exercises correctly, lead you toward your fitness goals, and help you achieve overall health. A trainer can be instrumental in preventing injuries by showing you proper workout techniques, and identifying techniques to avoid. Your trainer also should help you feel comfortable with the free weights, machines, and other workout equipment, thereby giving you the confidence to go to the gym on your own.

Besides helping you with equipment, your trainer should motivate and encourage you by making you accountable. Your trainer also should carefully watch, or "spot," you to protect you from injury. Since you'll be paying for the trainer's time and service, the trainer should be able to block out all distractions when working with you.

Before you hire a trainer, check credentials. Be certain the trainer looks the part and plays the part. Is the trainer a good example? Does the trainer have a good physique and follow a healthy lifestyle? Look for trainers who practice what they preach.

Finally, your trainer should be able to design a program that's right for you—not just a copy of what the trainer does. The next chapter includes helpful training suggestions that can work for everyone.

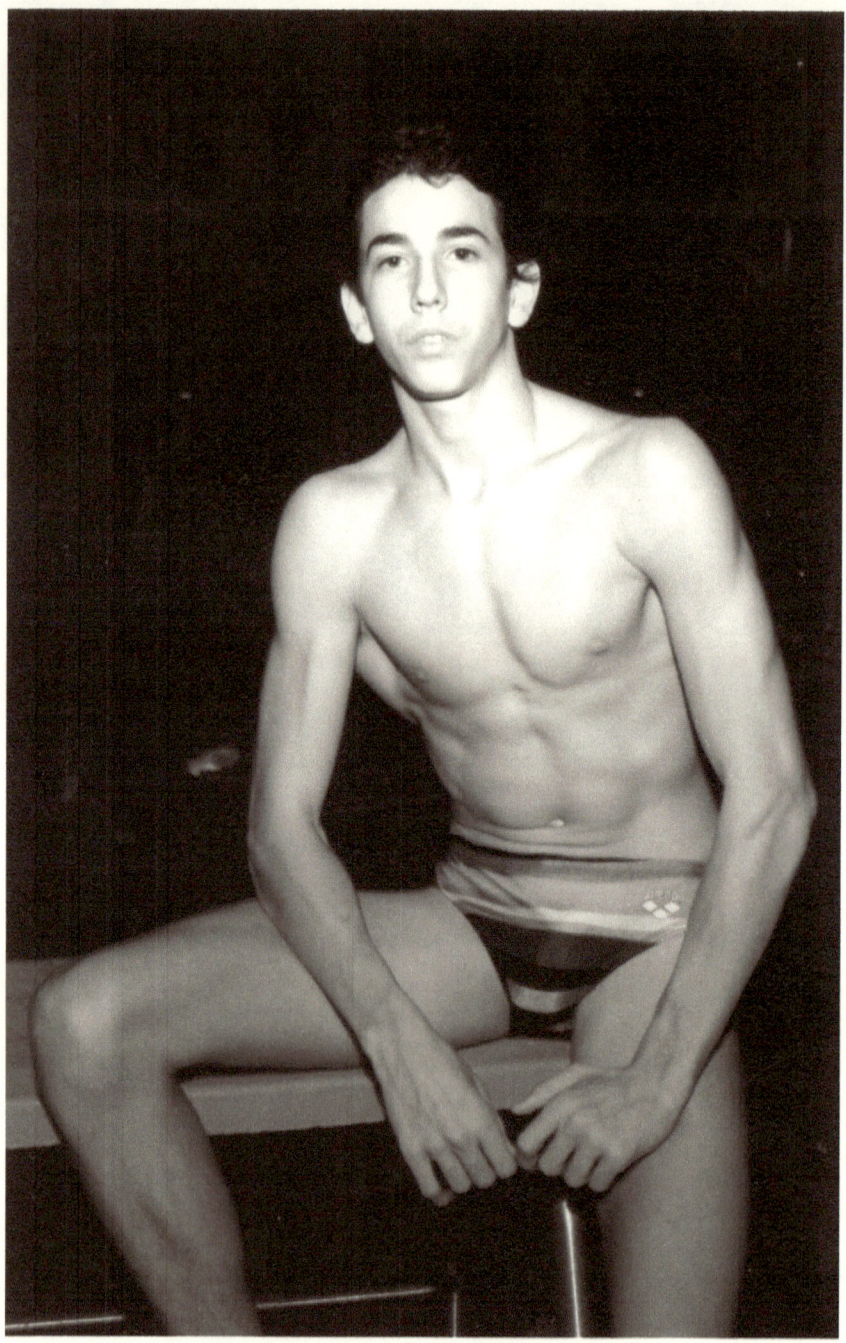

The skinny kid in high school, 1985

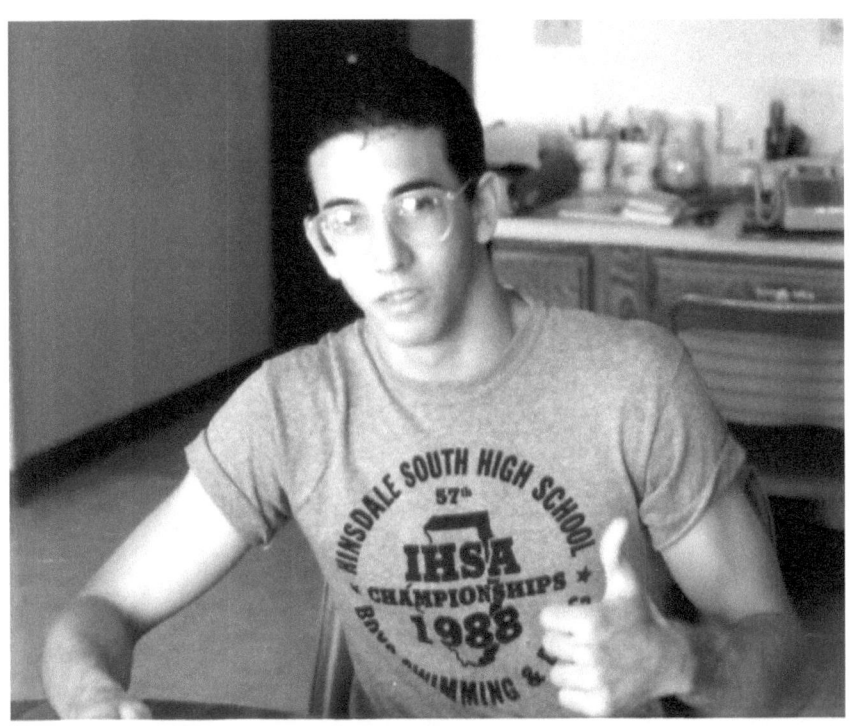

A year before I started seriously training, 1988

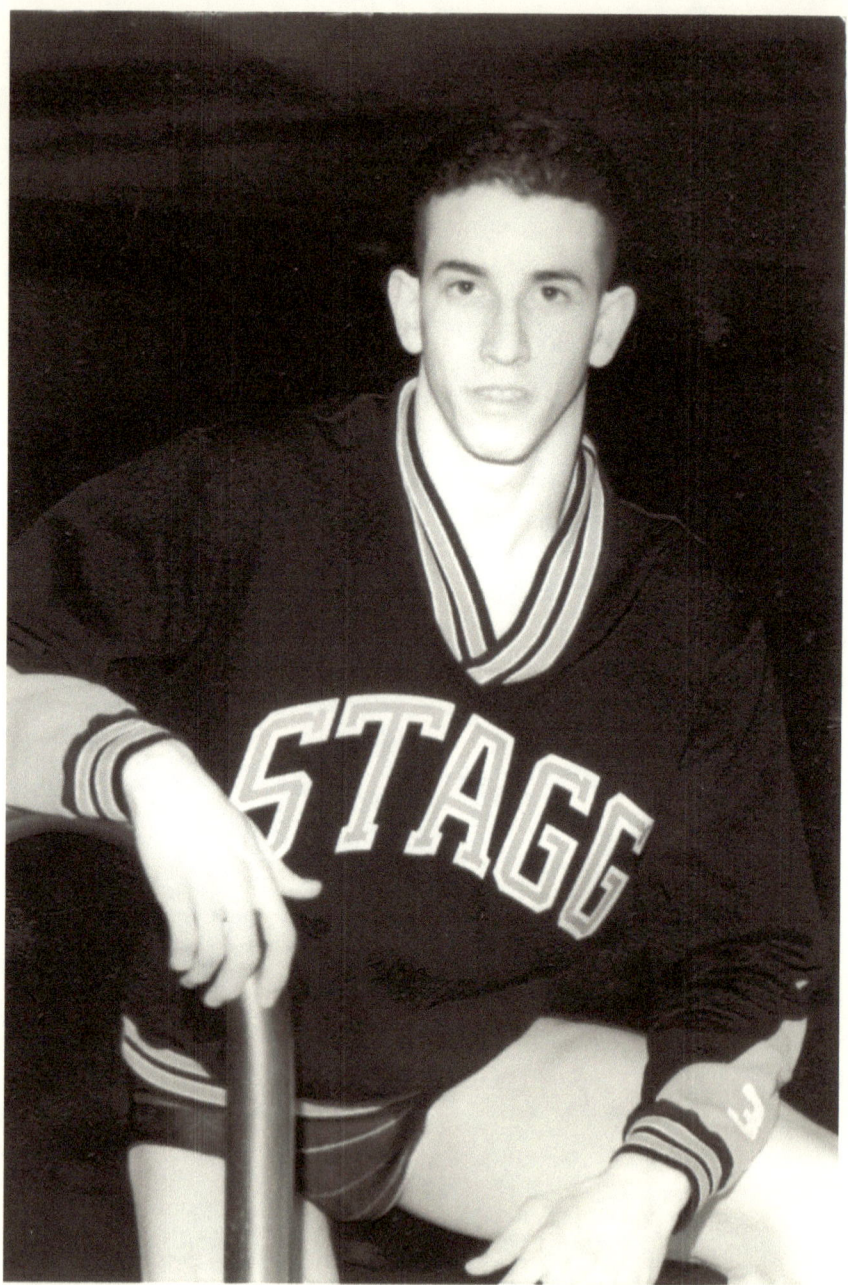

My senior year as a swimmer at Amos Alonzo Stagg High School, 1988

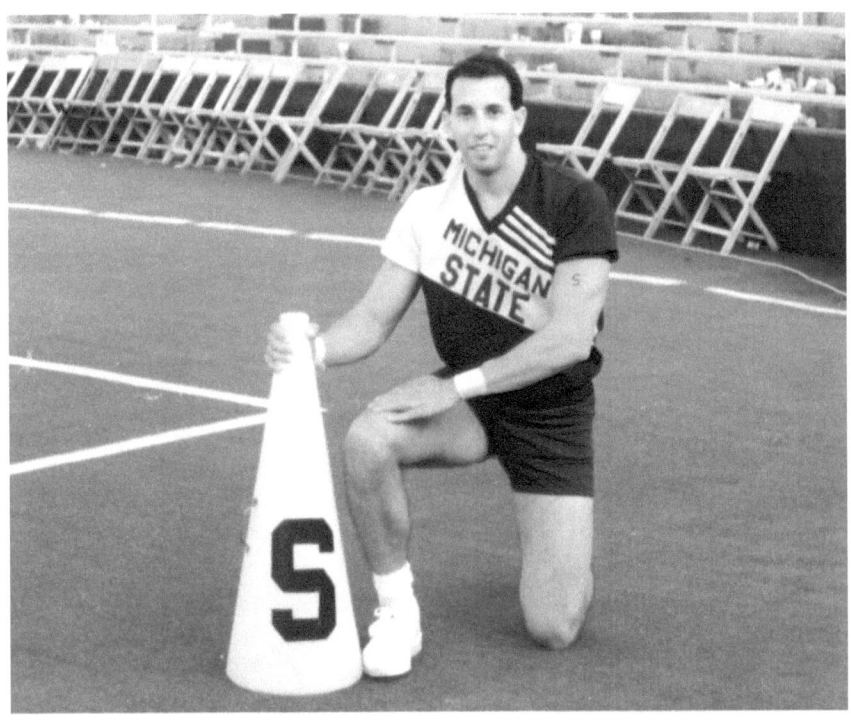

My cheerleading days at Michigan State, 1992

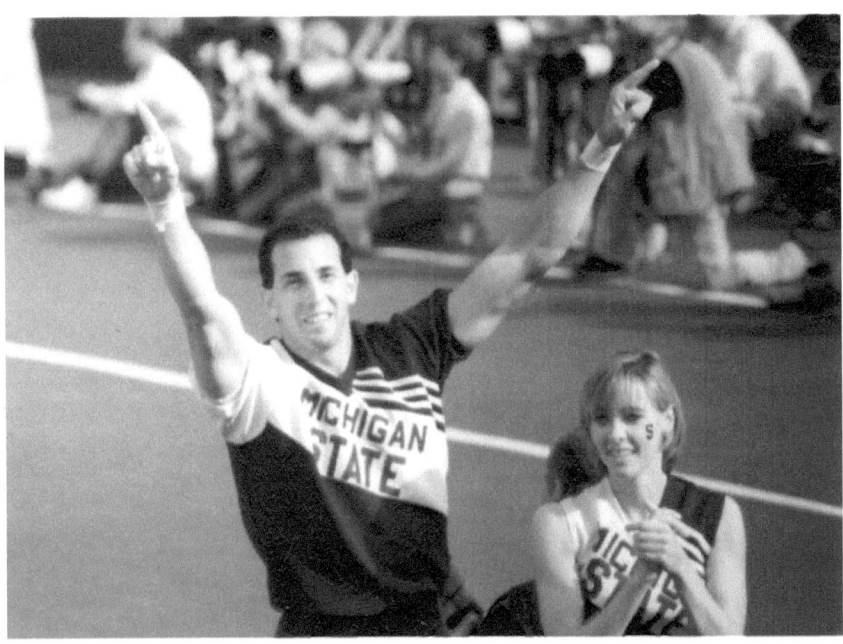

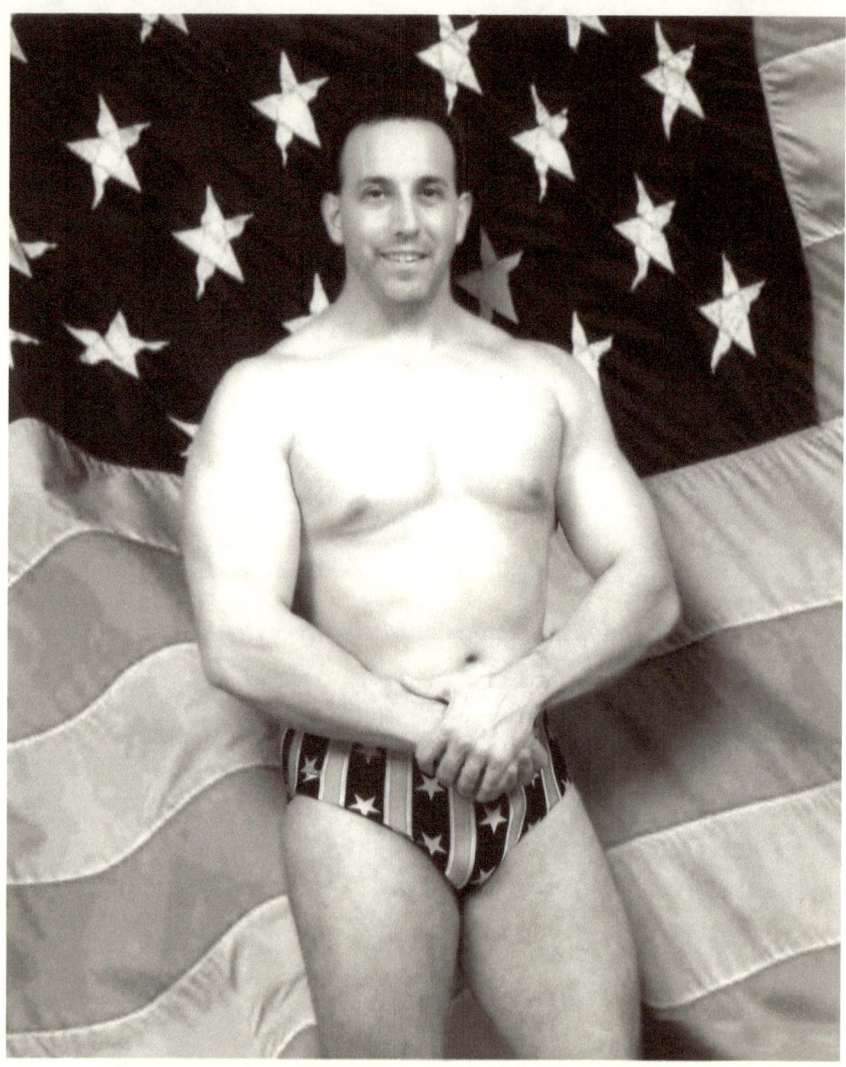

*Here is when I was overweight, smooth and on
the "opposite end of the spectrum", 2004*

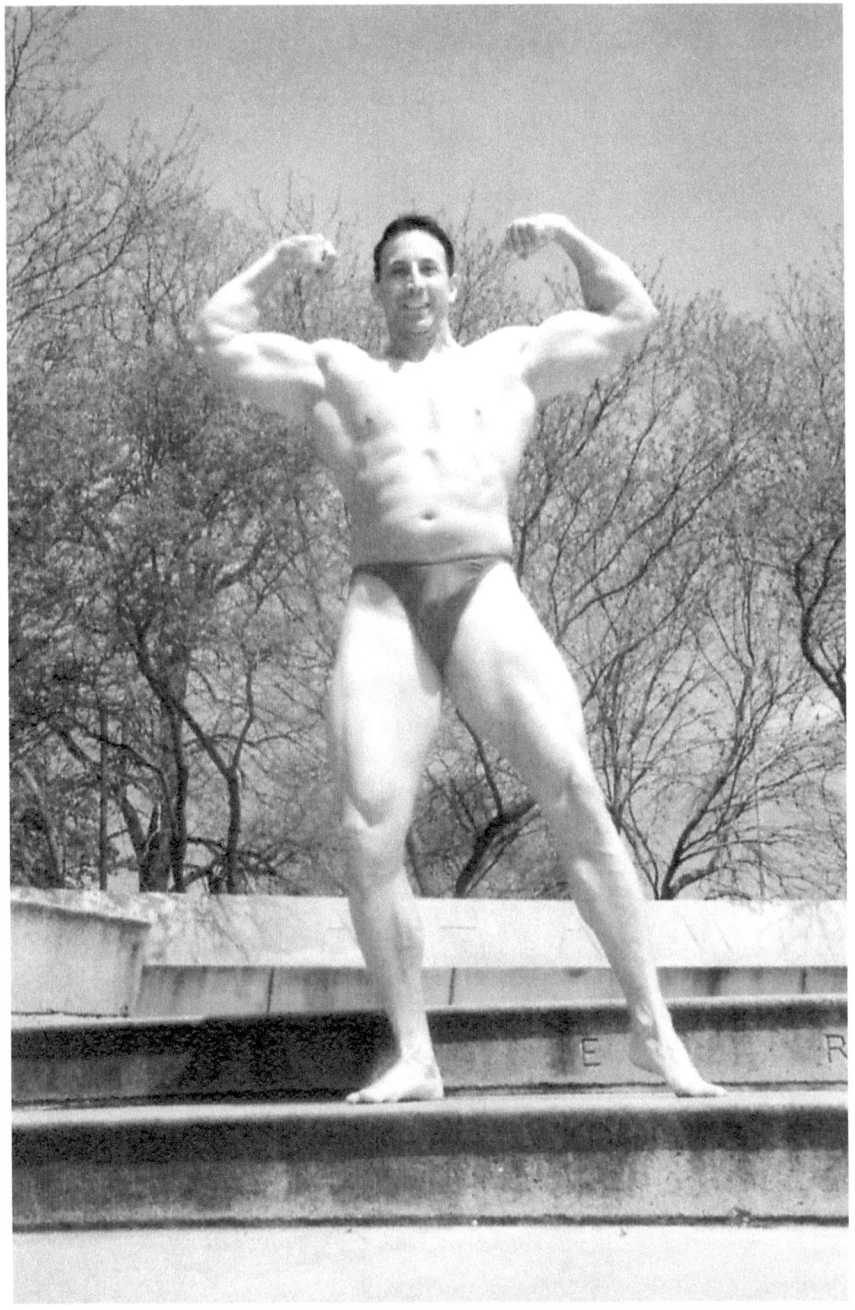

Doing a photo shoot in my off-season shape at 243 pounds, 2007

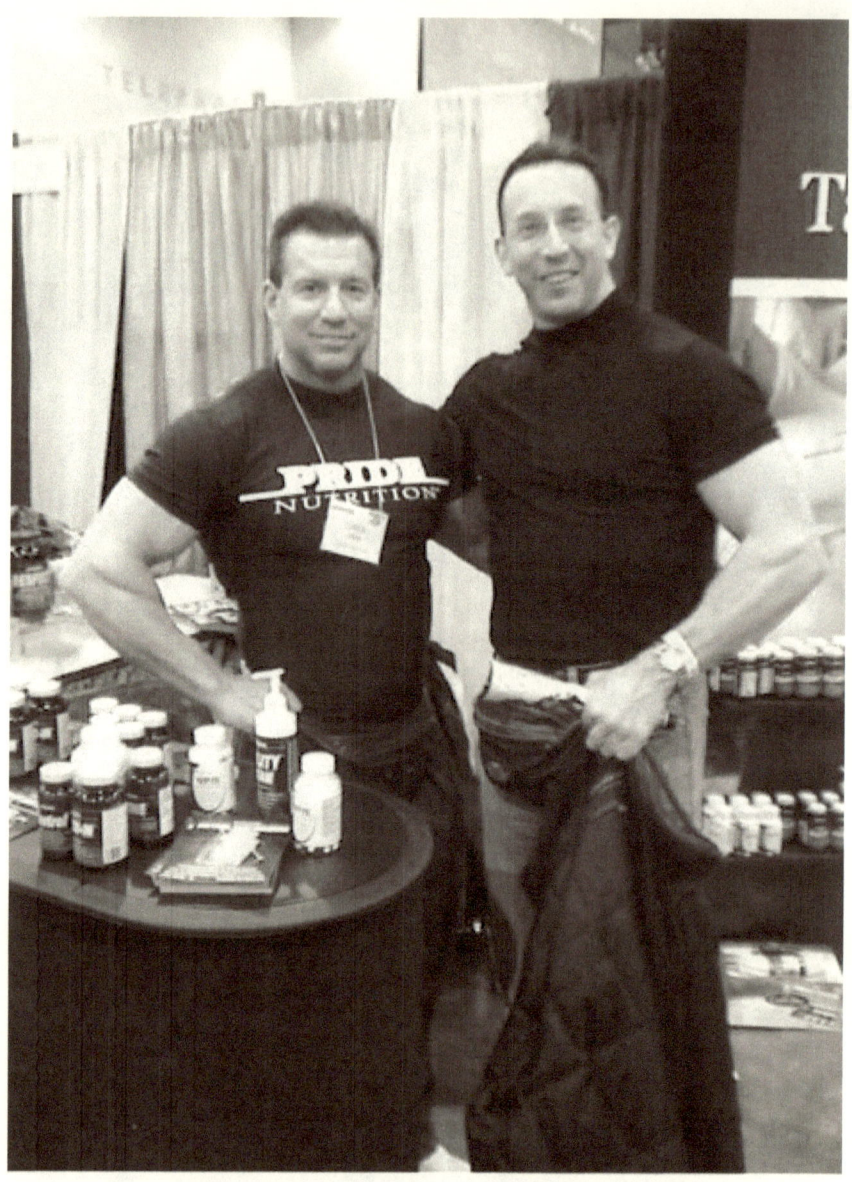

*Me with my mentor, USA Gym owner and
IFBB Pro Chuck Sanow, 2006*

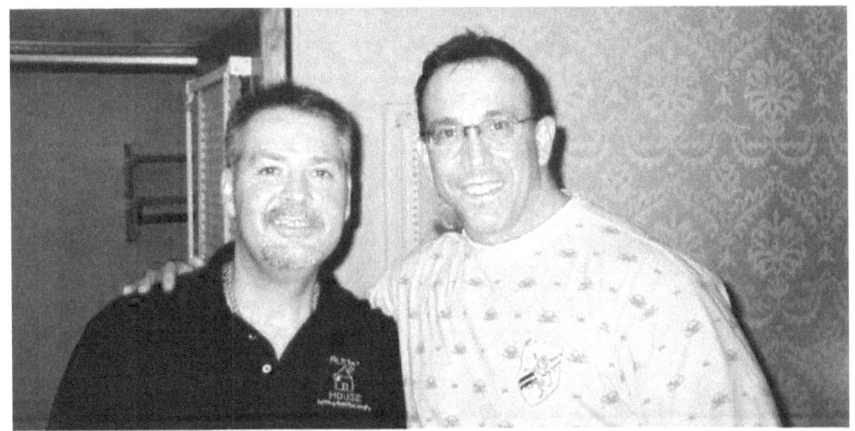

Me with Juan "Mr. Karate" Hernandez, a great guy and friend, 2007

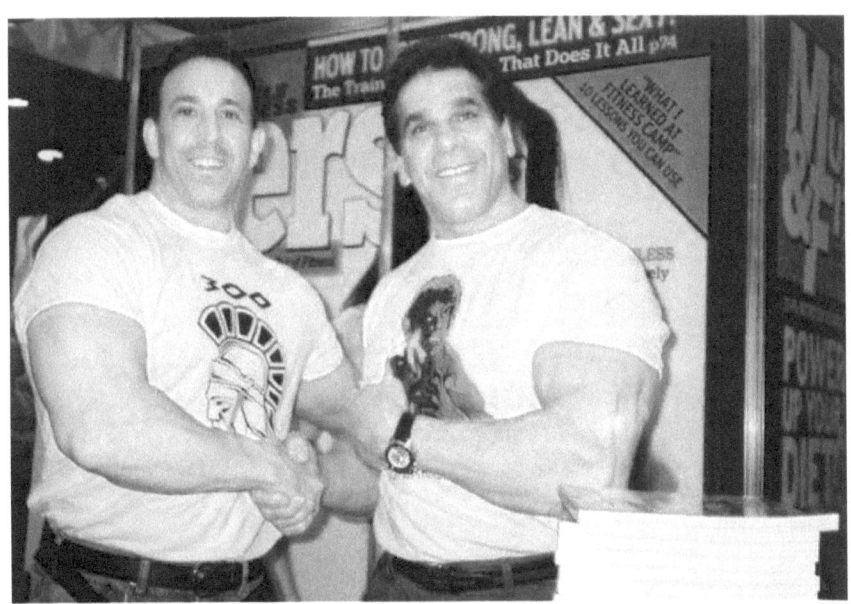

Lou Ferrigno was a big inspiration growing up. It was an honor meeting him at the Arnold Schwarzenegger Classic Expo, 2008

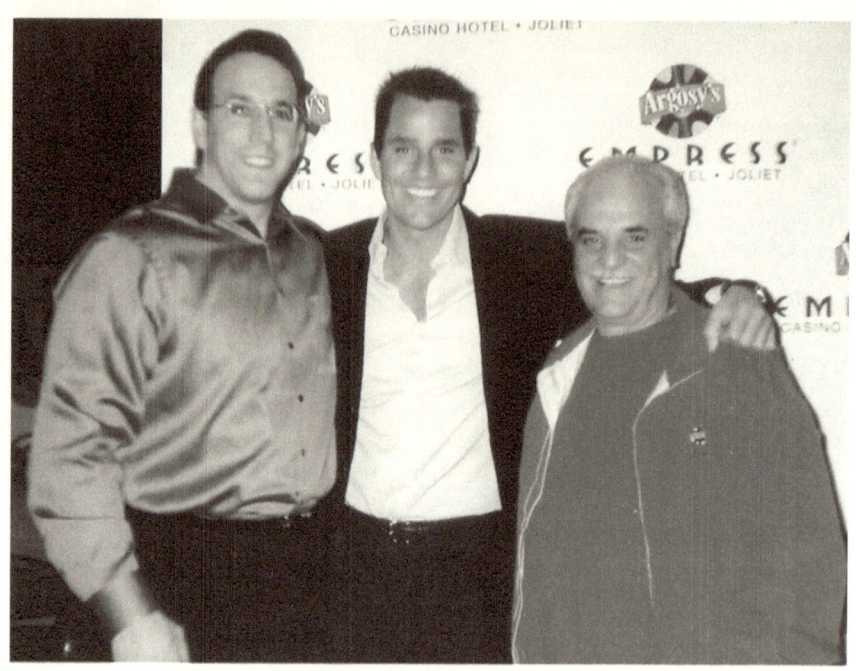

*My friend from the old neighborhood, Sam Di Franco.
He introduced me to Bill Rancic, winner of Donald
Trump's first season of The Apprentice, 2005*

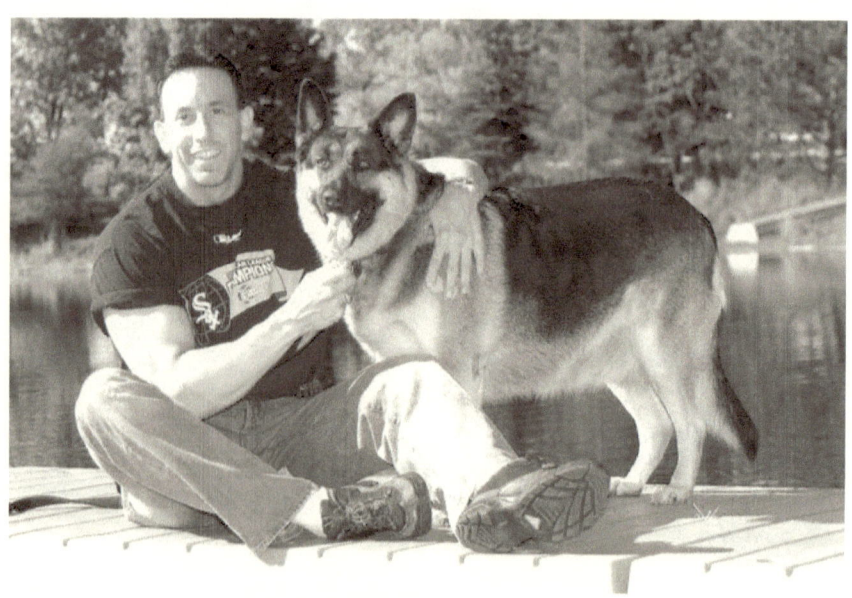

The author with Roxy.

CHAPTER 5:
PROGRAM DESIGN SUGGESTIONS FOR EVERYONE

During my twenty-five years of training and athletics, I've been confronted with a variety of reasons to work out. When I was thin, I wanted to gain weight and build muscle mass. When I became an athlete, I needed to increase my strength, improve my cardiovascular conditioning, and prevent injuries. When I competed in different sports, I needed my training to be sport-specific. My programs were designed to work the muscles for a particular sport, whether it be martial arts, college cheerleading, or bodybuilding. And, when I suffered an injury, I had to adjust my training for rehabilitation of the injury.

Now, as a competitive bodybuilder, I train to gain muscle mass when I am not competing—when I'm in my "off-season." But no matter whether I am off-season or in competition mode, I always train, focusing on conditioning, muscle tone, and shape. I do ample cardiovascular work to maintain the most important muscle in my body: the heart muscle. My training also helps me reduce and manage stress. Even for non-athletes—and perhaps especially for business professionals—working out can help in dealing with everyday stress.

Following are workout designs and principles that apply to a wide range of fitness goals. Whether you're a "Starter," a "Regular Exerciser/Maintainer," or a "Weight Reducer," there's information here to help you. I've also included suggestions for bodybuilders preparing for competition, and I share some of my favorite mass-building techniques that can give your muscles the shock they need to become thicker and fuller.

The Starter Program

Everyone is a starter at some point. I don't like to use the term "beginner." "Starter" is more of an action word. Before any star athletes became starting players on their teams or reached the top of their sports, they were "starters."

When new clients begin their fitness journeys, I often see in them a sense of awkwardness in going to the gym for the first time. When I see that awkwardness in their body language, I remind them that I, and every professional athlete, had to start somewhere. To ease the tension, I often share my own experience of the awkward feeling I had the first time I walked into a gym. Sometimes I show new clients a picture of myself when I was skinny, and assure them that they can change their bodies, too. I reinforce to my clients that, just like me, they must work out consistently, get to the gym regularly, and stay focused. That's the only way to see results. The key ingredient: patience. I was patient for ten years before I entered my first bodybuilding competition.

If you're a starter, you need to slowly ease into a workout program. Many starters have been living a sedentary lifestyle, are overweight, or are recovering from an illness or injury. Whatever your situation, I advise every starter to first consult with and get clearance from your physician before you begin any training program. Your physician should let you and your trainer know which exercises you should or should not perform.

As a starter, you should begin training with low-intensity cardio and light weights. Your muscles will need at least three to four weeks to get acclimated to weight training and aerobic exercise. Once your cardiovascular fitness increases and your muscles adapt to the weights, you should gradually increase the intensity and weight.

Here are some guidelines for a starter program:

- Train 2 to 3 days per week.

- Perform 15 to 25 minutes of cardio, starting at low intensity.

- Cardio should begin with 15 minutes at 65 percent of your target heart rate. Gradually increase by 5 minutes as cardiovascular endurance increases.

- Lift light to medium weights.

- Do 15 to 20 repetitions, 3 sets of each exercise.

- Actively train 30 to 40 minutes per workout, including both weight training and cardio training.

- Rest 2 to 3 minutes between sets.

THE REGULAR EXERCISER, OR "MAINTAINER"

If you're a regular exerciser, you train consistently to maintain or improve your physique. As a regular or "maintainer," you're primarily a self-motivated person who understands the importance of staying fit and healthy. Your time in the gym is habitual. It's just one of your everyday tasks, like brushing your teeth to maintain good dental health. There is nothing to think about; going to the gym or engaging in physical activity comes naturally.

However, if you're in the maintenance phase, you run the risk of hitting a plateau. A plateau can be discouraging, because you see no visible changes in your physique. Plateaus happen when your muscles become adapted to the exercise, so the result is only minimum muscle stimulation and recruitment of muscle fibers. Continuing to use the same exercises and the same weight does not contribute to the growth and development of muscle. If you're stuck in a plateau, you can become bored with your workouts and no longer adhere to your program.

Here are some guidelines to help maintainers improve their fitness levels and break through plateaus. The object is to avoid boredom and continue in your fitness journey:

- Train 3 times per week.

- Lift moderate to heavy weights, increasing the weight on each set.

- Do a minimum of 3 sets of 10 to 12 repetitions each.

- Rest 1 to 3 minutes between sets.

- Change the exercises for each body part.

- Perform cardiovascular activity for 30 to 45 minutes.

WEIGHT LOSS/WEIGHT MANAGEMENT

Most of the inquiries I get are from people who are interested in hiring a personal trainer because they're struggling with their weight. They deserve all the credit in the world for taking that first step to overcome their weight problem and make changes. I believe that diet is responsible for 85 percent of any weight loss, weight management, or significant changes to your physique that you achieve. As I noted earlier, I am not a dietitian or nutritionist, so I'm only able to offer tips for the workout portion of a weight loss/weight management program. I have seen people lose weight, then face the real challenge of keeping the weight off. Here are some recommendations to help you succeed:

- Train 5 to 6 times per week.

- Lift light weights, gradually increasing with strength.

- Perform 1-3 sets of 8 to 12 repetitions for 6 to 10 total exercises.

- Do 45 to 60 minutes of low-intensity cardio, starting gradually and staying within 40 to 50 percent of your target heart rate.

OTHER WORKOUT ROUTINES

CIRCUIT TRAINING

I was first introduced to circuit training in the mid-1980s, when I was on the high school cross-country team. After completing a long run, the team would go to the weight room to lift weights. When I went to the weight room, my intention was to put some muscle on this skinny frame, even though cross-country is an endurance sport. After doing a few sets of arm curls, the girls' cross-country coach would ask the boys if we wanted to do the circuit. Being the open minded person that I am, I decided to give circuit training a try.

We did the circuit by starting at one exercise station, working there for 30 seconds, then moving to the neighboring station. For example, I might start with the chest station and work my pectorals, then move to the triceps station and do triceps pushdowns. The girls' coach had a stopwatch and would yell, "Time!" after each set. Between sets, we would rest briefly before starting the next station. I have to admit that I enjoyed this type of routine. I got a good workout, and I was exhausted afterwards.

Circuit training enhances muscular endurance, muscular strength, and aerobic conditioning. After doing circuit training on and off over the years, I have experienced these benefits. Circuit training is used in sport-specific training; I used it during my years of cross county and 5K runs, and nine years of competitive swimming. Here are some of the components for circuit training:

- Select workstations for each body part.
- Do as many repetitions as possible; aim for at least 12 to 15.
- Rest either between exercises or upon completion of all exercise stations.
- Rest 30 to 60 seconds between exercise stations, or at completion of all work stations before repeating the circuit.

TOTAL BODY ROUTINE

The total body routine is something I do in hotel gyms when I'm on the road. It's ideal for maintainers. I recommend it for my clients who have extremely busy schedules or who cannot see me on a consistent or weekly basis. A total body routine trains every body part in an hour, just to stimulate the muscles. Here are the components of a total body program, indicating which parts are targeted by each component:

- Do push exercises for the upper body: chest, triceps, and shoulders.

- Then perform lower-body push exercises: legs (quadricep-dominant exercises).

- Next, perform pull exercises for the upper body: back, biceps.

- Then do lower-body pull exercises: legs (hip-dominant exercises).

- Perform 3 to 4 sets, 10 to 15 repetitions each.

THE BODYBUILDER

If you're a bodybuilder, you're constantly striving for continual body transformation. Training for bodybuilding is geared toward building bigger, harder muscles. The goal is to achieve an aesthetically pleasing look by having a symmetrical and proportionate physique.

When bodybuilders compete on the contest stage, they're under the close scrutiny of a panel of judges. The judges compare the competitors' physiques and body parts against one another through mandatory poses. Each bodybuilder wants to be bigger and harder than the other competitors.

For seven years, I have competed as an all-natural, drug-free bodybuilder. I want to prove that it is possible to gain muscle mass naturally, without anabolic steroids, growth hormone, or other drugs. I want be "living proof" that it can be done.

To compete in bodybuilding competition, you must have a determined mindset and self-discipline. You also must keep everything on schedule—training, proper rest, diet—and you must keep your stress level as low as possible. During my off-season, I lift heavy and strive for adequate blood flow to the muscle groups I'm working. I make sure I'm struggling on that last set and the final few repetitions.

Here are some guidelines for a good bodybuilding program:

- Train 5 to 6 times per week.

- Work 1 body part per day.

- Rest and recover for 48 hours for each body part.

- Perform 4 to 5 sets of each exercise.

- Do repetitions of 12–10–10–8–6, increasing the weight for each set.

- Rest for 1 to 3 minutes after each set.

BIG LEE'S WEEKLY TRAINING ROUTINE

I've been doing this routine since June 2006. Ever since I adopted it, I've seen a positive change in my physique. This routine allows me to work one body part per day, solely focusing on that body part and working it to fatigue. Training to fatigue means that I go to the point where I can't lift the weight at my last set and last repetition. When I'm done with a workout, I'm getting "the pump" as the blood flows speedily to the muscles I just worked. This routine also prevents overtraining, which hinders muscle growth, and it allows plenty of time for muscles to rest, repair, and grow. And if I miss a day, I can make it up on the weekend.

My routine follows this schedule:

- Monday: chest

- Tuesday: back

- Wednesday: legs

- Thursday: shoulders
- Friday: arms

In addition, I follow these guidelines:

- Train abdominals and calves every day.
- Perform cardio for 30 minutes per day.
- Stretch between sets and at the end of the workout.

Off-Season

During my off-season, I go heavy and do a lot of super-setting to get that pump through working my muscles to total fatigue. The blood pumps rapidly to the muscles, and the muscle expansion is noticeable. For the muscles to continue growing, I must supply them with proper nutrients and rest. Doing it naturally takes longer, but the muscle will stay with me for a lifetime if I train consistently.

Remember this: when you're in the gym, you're tearing down; when you're resting and eating, you're building. It's important to eat immediately after a grueling workout to get the proper nutrients to the muscles. This allows them to grow, and increases the number of muscle fibers.

Contest Preparation

Twelve weeks prior to a competition, I begin my diet and make changes in my workout routine. I start doing cardio twice a day for 30 minutes to get my body in "fat-burning mode." The increase in cardio coupled with the strict diet cuts out the excess body fat and water that I hold in the off-season.

I also change the amount of weight I lift. During contest prep, I train with moderately heavy weights. When the contest is about five weeks away, I change to lighter weights and more repetitions. This allows me to burn more fat and calories to further define my physique.

COMPETITIVE BODYBUILDING: ON STAGE

When bodybuilders are on stage, underneath the hot lights in front of the judges, they are rated on the following criteria:

- Overall presentation and total package
- Size: muscular development of each body part
- Symmetry: balance and proportion of the physique
- Muscularity: lack of body fat and big presence of muscle definition and striation

RELAXED POSITION

Backstage at a bodybuilding contest in the "pump-up room" is fascinating. You'll see competitors "pumping up" with dumbbells and barbells, or with the few benches available. Competitors will oil each other and pump up with tubing before an expeditor calls each weight class to get lined up and ready to go on stage. When competitors are lined up backstage, it's usually dead silent until they come out and do their required mandatory poses.

When the competitors are called out to the stage, they first line up shoulder-to-shoulder in the "relaxed position" before the judges. In this round, the judges are looking for proportion, shape, and balance in the relaxed position. The head judge will command the competitors to do quarter turns in the relaxed position. Here are some important tips to help you correctly do the quarter turns:

- Face your head the same direction that your feet are facing.
- Keep your hands at your sides.
- Avoid twisting.
- Keep your feet flat.
- Place the right foot behind the heel and pivot the body while doing quarter turns.

MANDATORY POSES

Competitors are then directed to perform the mandatory poses. Judges assess muscle size, symmetry, and muscularity by comparing one competitor to another.

These are the mandatory poses:

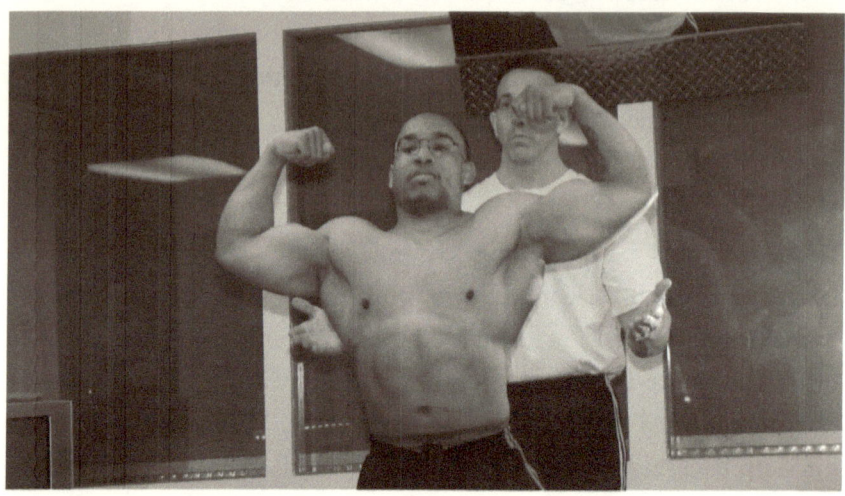

1. Front double bicep

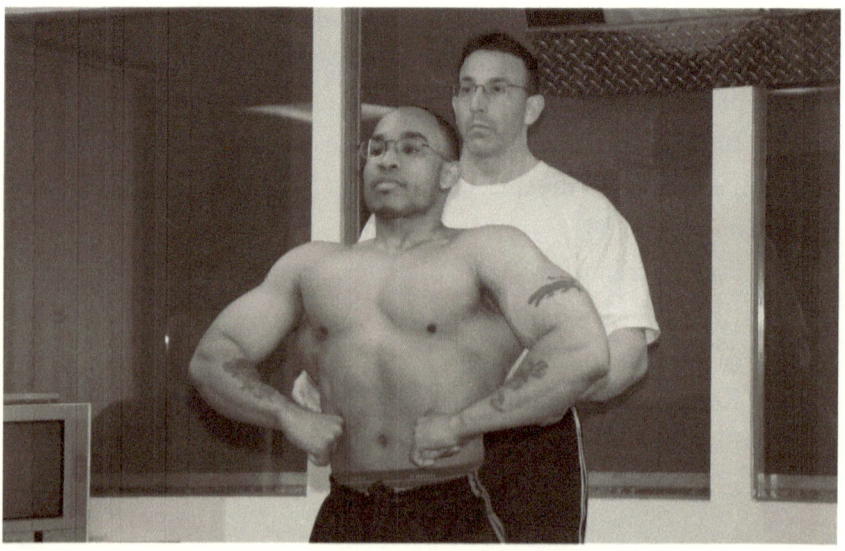

2. Front lat spread

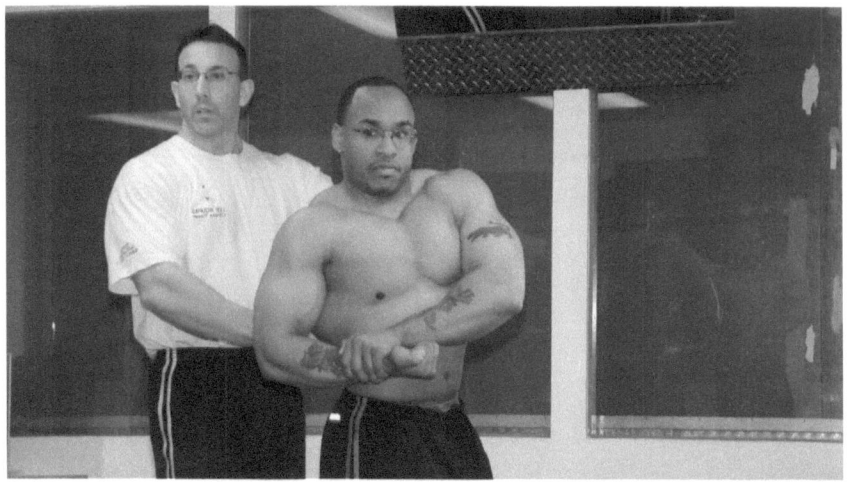

3. Side chest pose (either side)

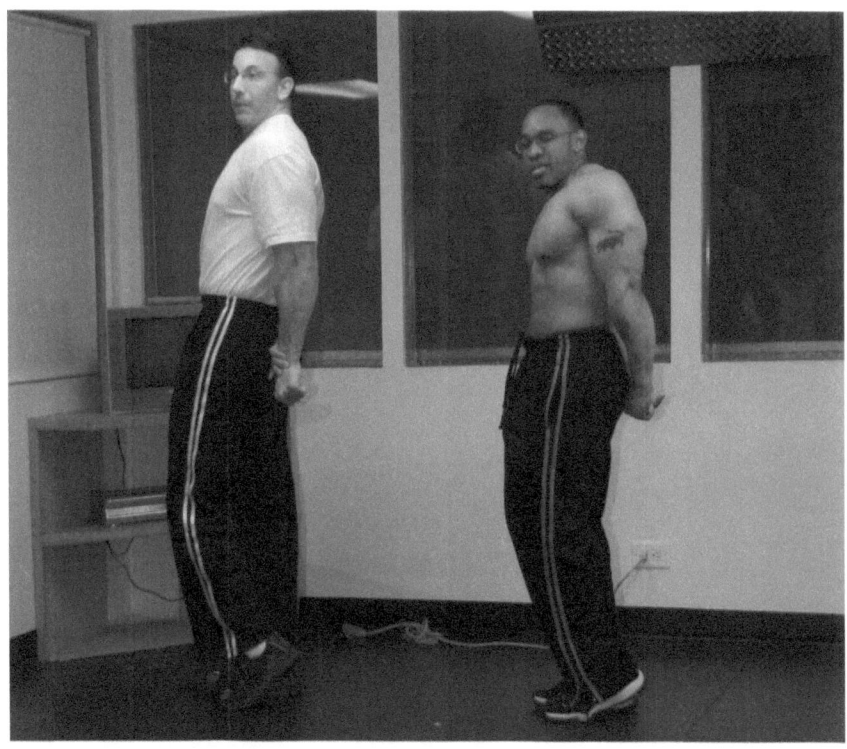

4. Side tricep (either side)

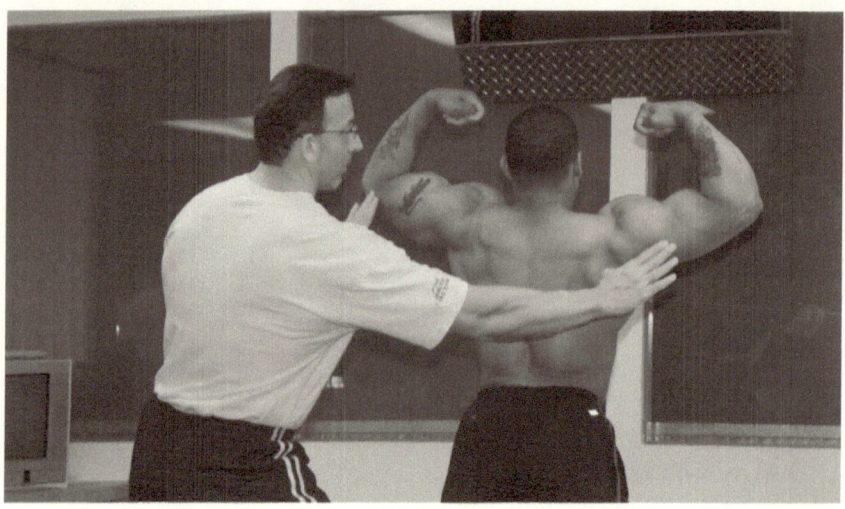

5. Back double bicep

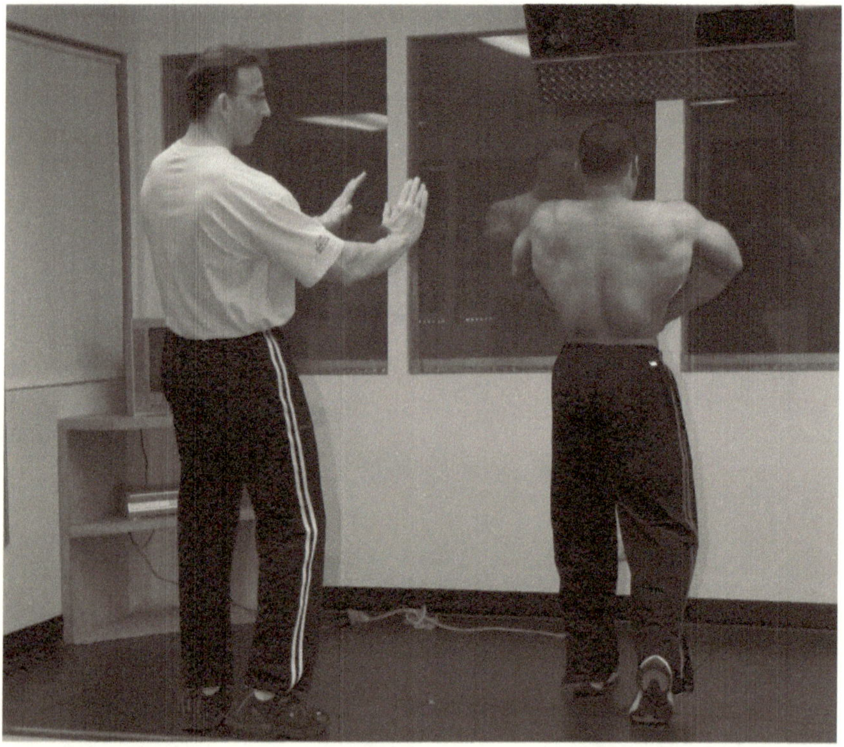

6. Rear lat spread

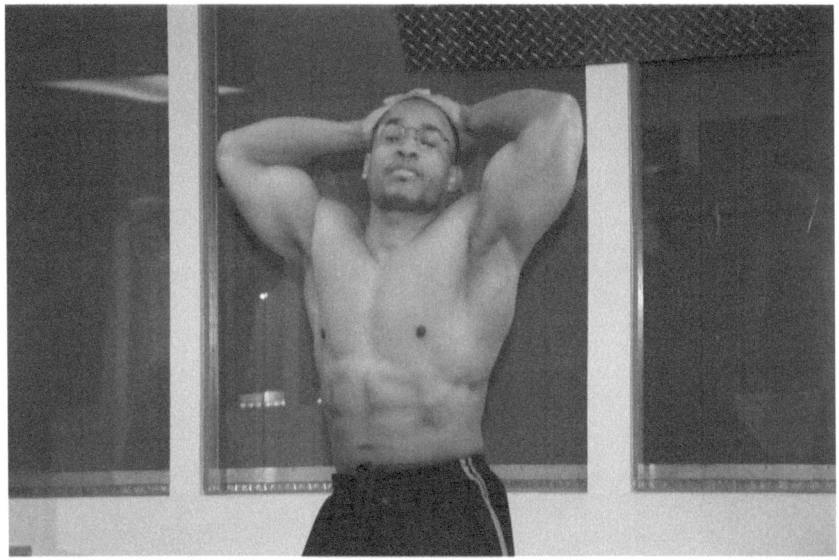

7. Abdominal pose

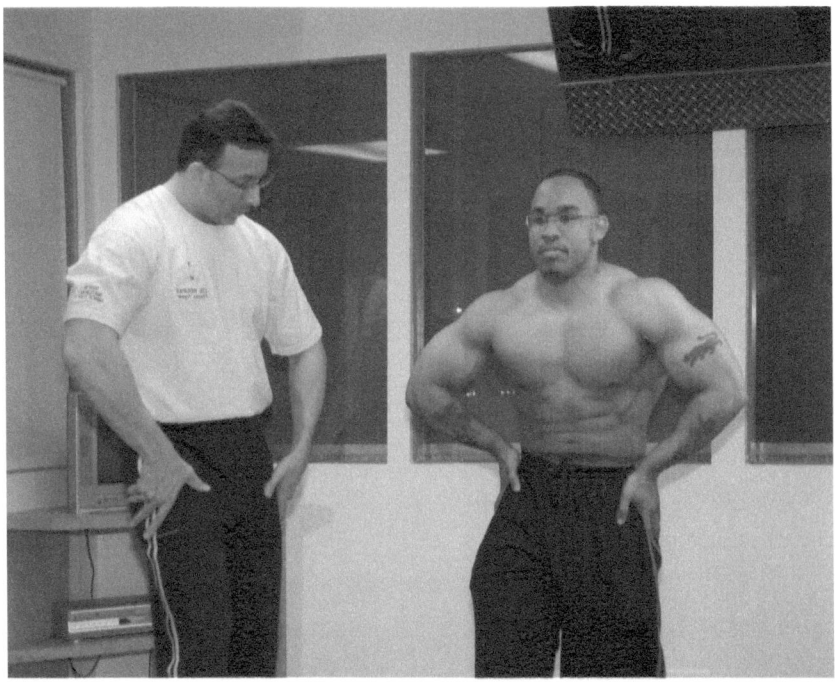

8. Most muscular

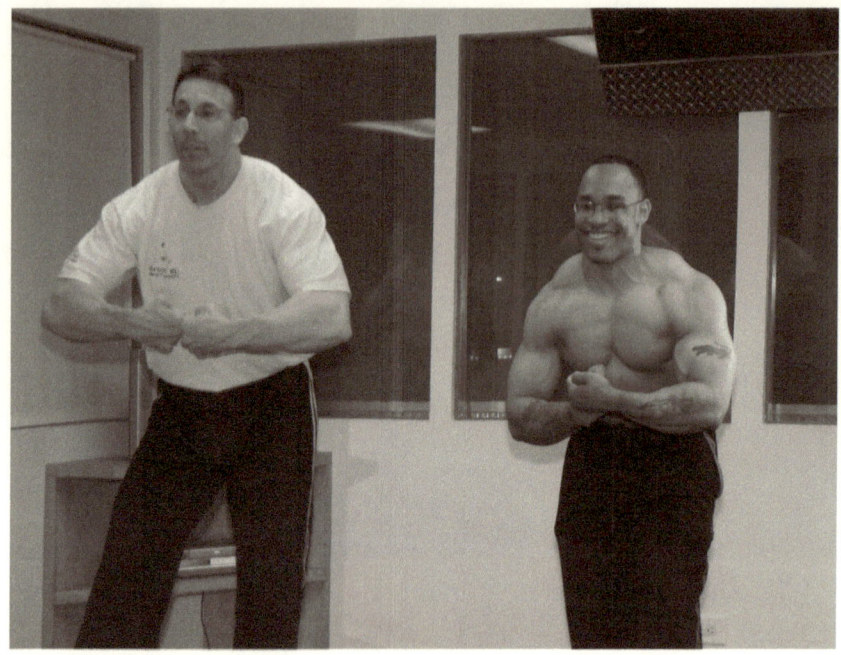

9. Crab Most Muscular (men only)

OTHER MASS-BUILDING
WORKOUT TECHNIQUES

DOWN THE RACK

I will never forget when Chuck Sanow introduced me to the "down-the-rack" technique. Chuck was taking me through an unbelievable arm workout using alternating dumbbell curls. He had me begin with a heavy weight that I was able to do comfortably for 6 to 8 repetitions. I would do as many repetitions as possible until failure; then, without rest, I would go "down the rack" and lift a weight that was five pounds lighter (alternatively, you can rest between weights). I do this technique until I can't do any more curls.

DROP SETS

I love doing drop sets! Begin with a weight that you can lift for 12 to 15 repetitions. Once you reach the point of failure, reduce the weight by half and try to complete 10 to 12 repetitions on the next set. Repeat this for 3 to 4 sets. On the last set, you should barely be able to lift an extremely light weight. If you cannot do the extremely light weight, you have done the drop sets correctly.

REST/PAUSE TECHNIQUE

I'm always looking for new ideas that can help break the monotony and improve the quality and effectiveness of a workout. One of those is the rest/pause technique, which can work muscle for substantial gains.

One of my arm workouts is the one-arm preacher curl. When I use the rest/pause technique, I do as many repetitions as I can until I hit the point of failure. I put the weight down, rest for 5 to 10 seconds, then pick the weight back up and crank out more repetitions to the point of failure. I do this for 3 to 4 sets.

SUPERSETS

Incorporating supersets into your workout gives the muscles a good "shock" for growth and development. Supersets also are good when you're short on time (thus eliminating the "I-have-no-time" excuse). There are days when I have appointments or business meetings, the gym is closing in an hour, and I must get a workout done. Instead of missing a workout, I do supersets.

You can use supersets to train the same or different muscle groups. It's especially useful with pushing exercises, such as exercises for chest and triceps. Begin with a weight that you can lift for 12 repetitions using good form. When you have completed one exercise, go immediately— without rest—to the next exercise. Increasing the weight on each set can bring the muscles to the point of total exhaustion.

CHAPTER 6:
WARMING UP, COOLING DOWN, AND STRETCHING

THE WARM-UP

Many people suffer workout-related or sports injuries because they fail to warm up sufficiently before engaging in activity. Warming up increases your metabolic rate, and it prepares the targeted muscles to be filled with blood and to be trained. Warming up also enables the cardiovascular system to increase blood flow to the muscles, supplying them with oxygen and other beneficial nutrients.

My warm-up consists of a 15-minute, low-intensity jog or run on the treadmill. This increases my body temperature and blood flow, and creates greater elasticity in my muscles and connective tissue. This, in turn, helps prevent soft tissue and muscle tears when I perform strenuous weight training.

After your muscles are warmed and ready to work, train the body part you want to train. Here are some additional tips:

- Aerobic activity should begin at low intensity.
- When performing the first set of an exercise, start with a light weight. This helps muscles to get adapted to the weight, and also allows you to practice good form.

THE COOL-DOWN

Cooling down after a workout is essential. When you're performing cardiovascular training, such as high-intensity aerobic activity, your arteries open wide to increase blood flow. If you stop suddenly, the sudden decrease in blood flow can cause blood pressure to plummet, resulting in dizziness or fainting. Blood also can pool in your legs and may clot; these blood clots can ultimately lead to stroke, especially in older people.

When you're ready to cool down, gradually start slowing the tempo and decreasing the intensity of your current activity. It's important to keep moving, though at a slower place, to maintain the blood flow to the brain and heart. Follow these tips:

- Cool down with aerobic exercise for two minutes, gradually lowering the intensity.
- Bring heart rate and breathing down to normal levels.

STRETCHING

Stretching should be done both before and after your workout. I recommend stretching after an easy warm-up. When your muscles are warmed up, they'll have an easier time loosening up. Stretching after a workout, especially after a cool-down, will elongate the muscles and assist in putting muscle fibers back in line. Stretching also can increase flexibility and prevent injuries. Here are some general guidelines for stretching:

- Stretching should be done for 5 to 10 minutes.
- Stretching should be gradual and should not hurt.
- Stretches should be held for 10 seconds.
- Avoid bouncing during a stretch.

STRETCHES FOR THE UPPER BODY

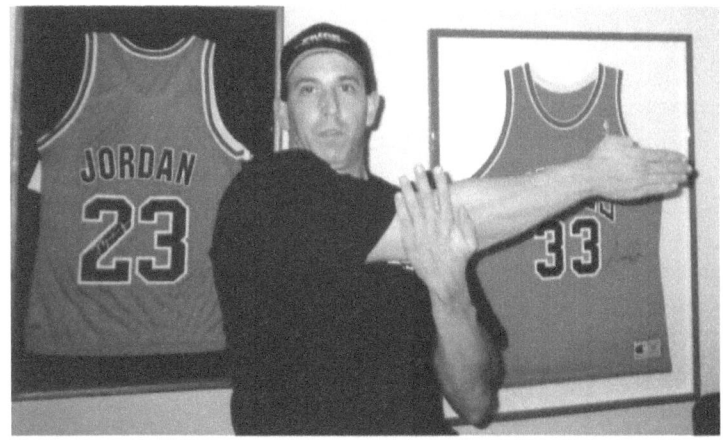

Shoulder Stretch (Posterior Deltoid)

Rotate your arm across your chest and pull above the elbow.

Arm Circles

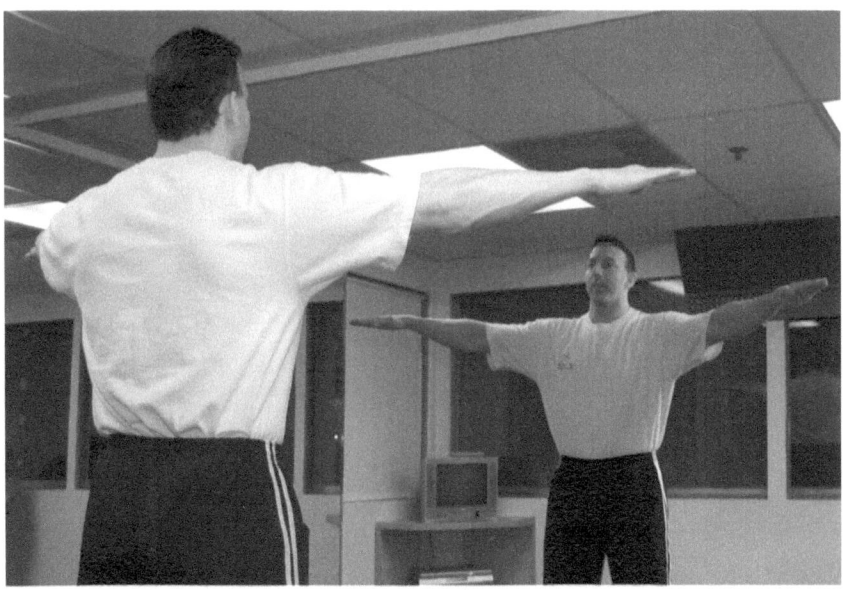

Hold arms straight out from your sides and begin moving them in a circular motion. Start with small circles, then increase the radius of the circles until your arms are circling as close to your ears as possible.

Chest Stretches

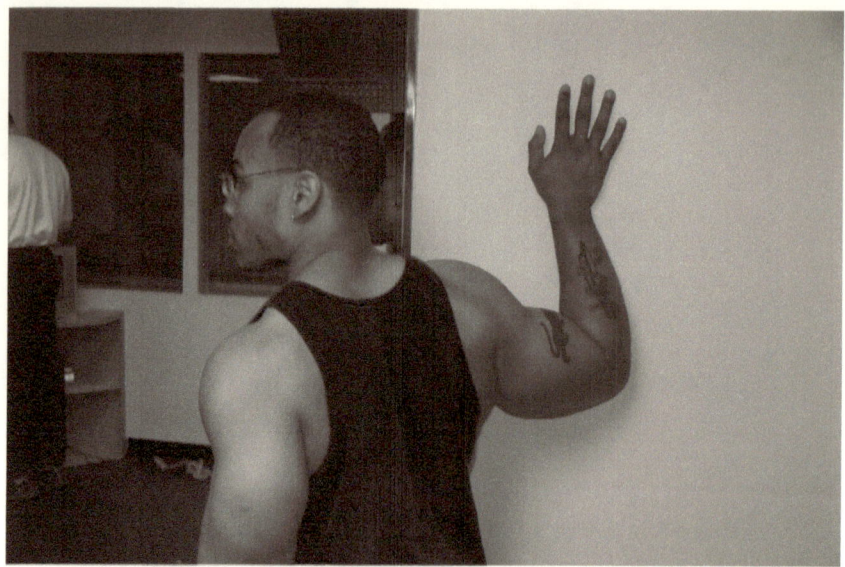

- Bend your elbow at a 90-degree angle, making the elbow even with your shoulder. Place your forearm and hand on the wall and turn your body counterclockwise.

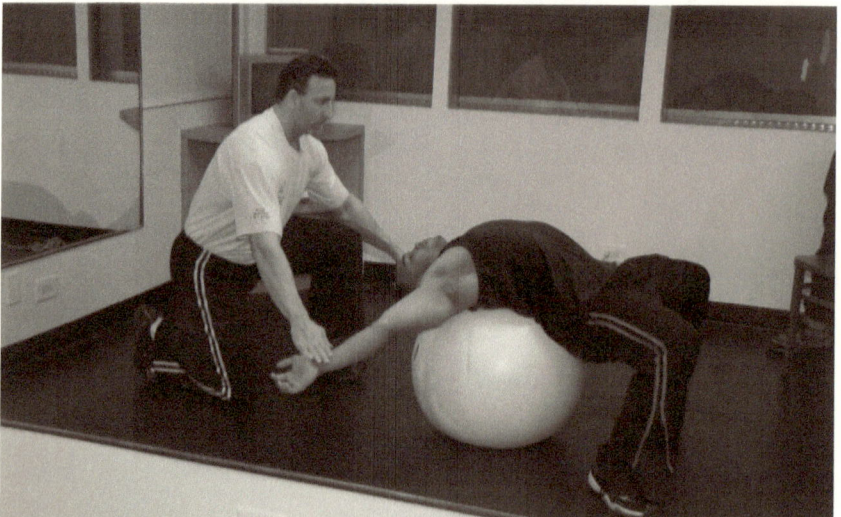

- Lie on an exercise ball with arms hanging straight to the side and open the chest, stretching your pectoral muscles.

Biceps and Anterior Deltoid Stretch

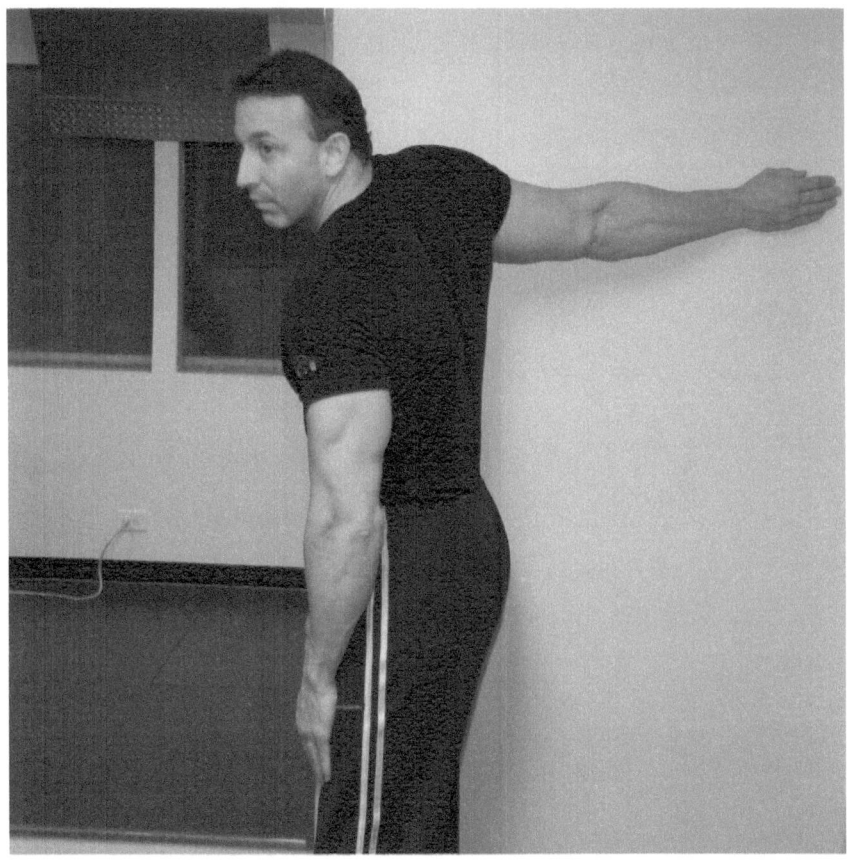

Straighten your arm against the wall,
and turn counter-clockwise.

Triceps Stretch

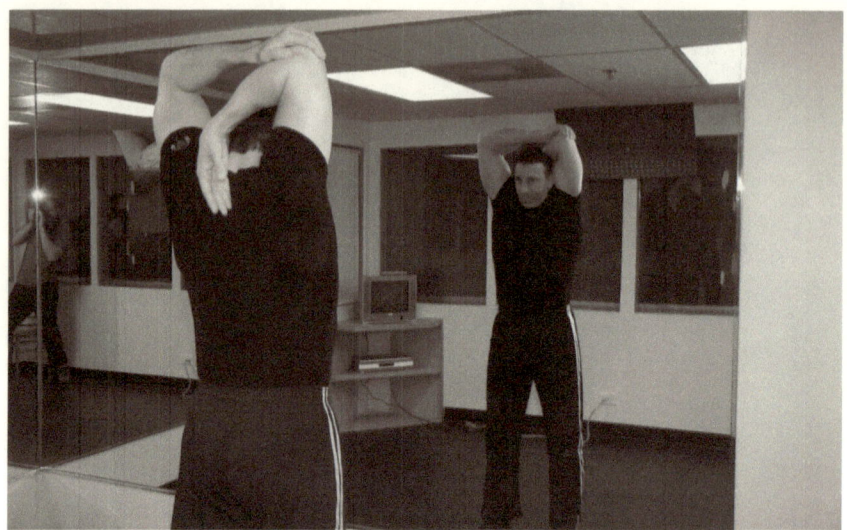

Bend your elbow, placing the arm over your head,
and use the opposite hand to pull the elbow back.

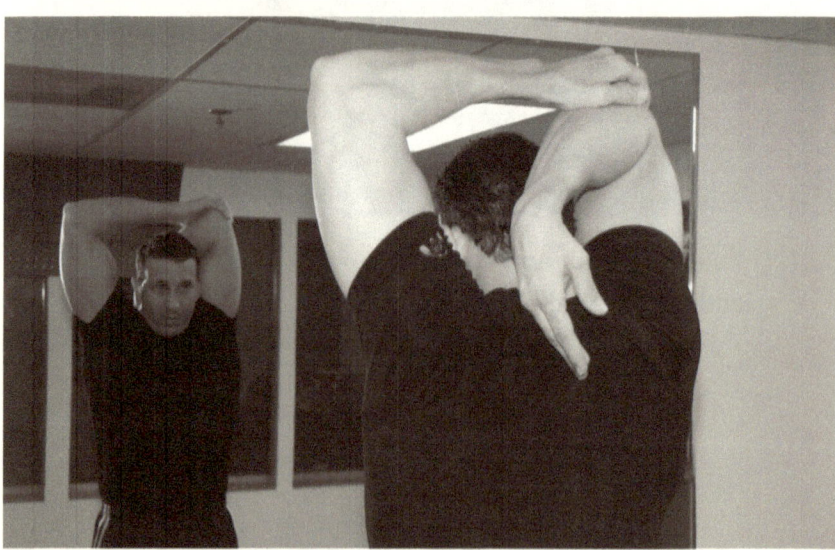

Back Stretch

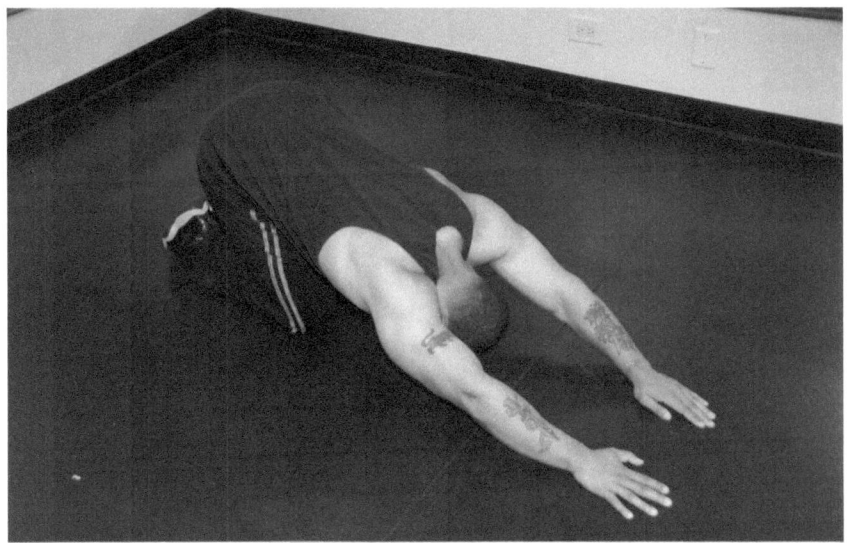

Place both hands above your head at shoulder width,
and push down with head between the arms.

Latissimus Stretch

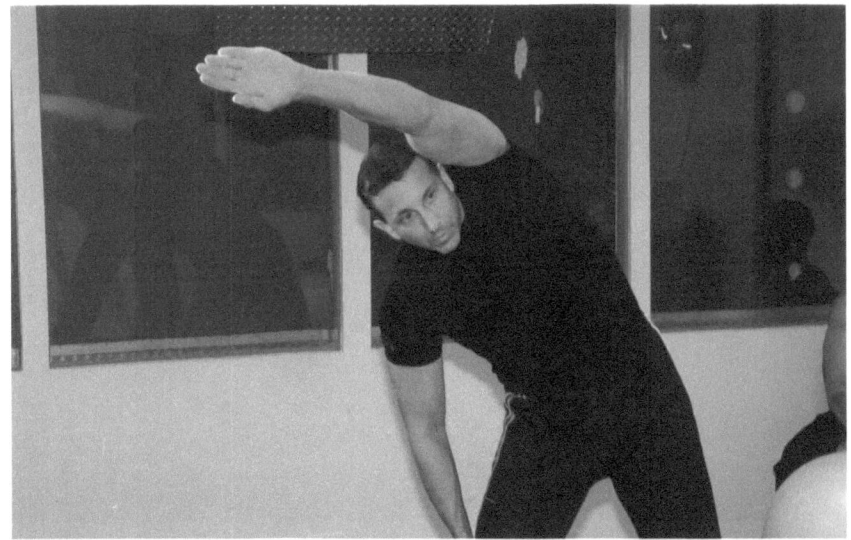

Lean to the side and extend your arm over your
head. Your bicep should touch your ear.

Lower- Back Stretch

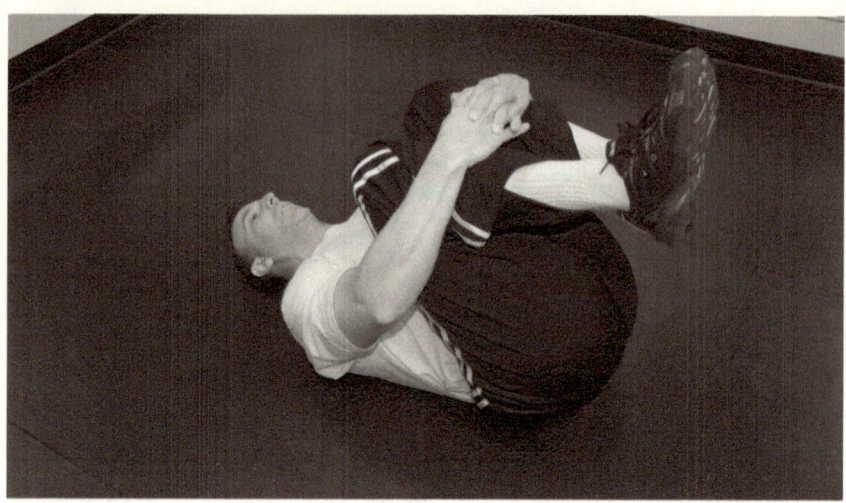

Lie on your back and gently pull your knees
toward your chest. You can pull one knee at
a time, or both knees simultaneously.

Abdominal Stretch

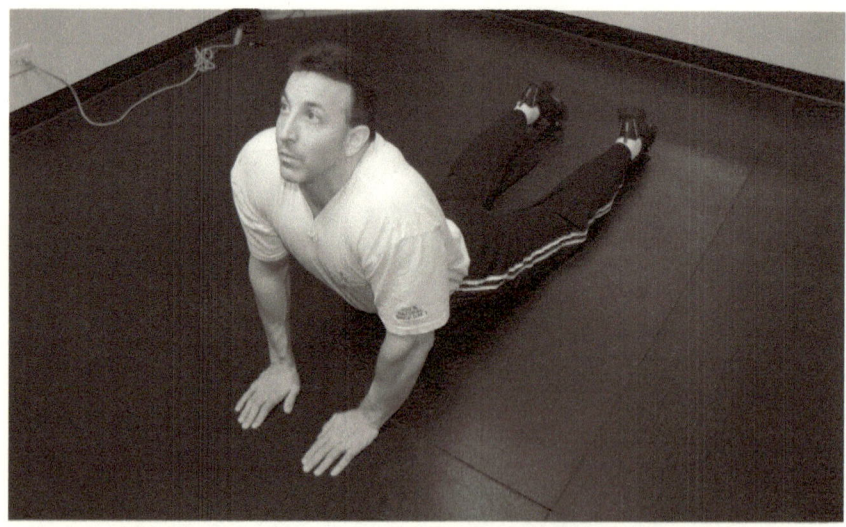

Lie down in a prone position on the floor and place
your hands under your chest. Push up into full
arm extension. Your head must be looking up.

Stretches for the Lower Body

Quadriceps Stretch

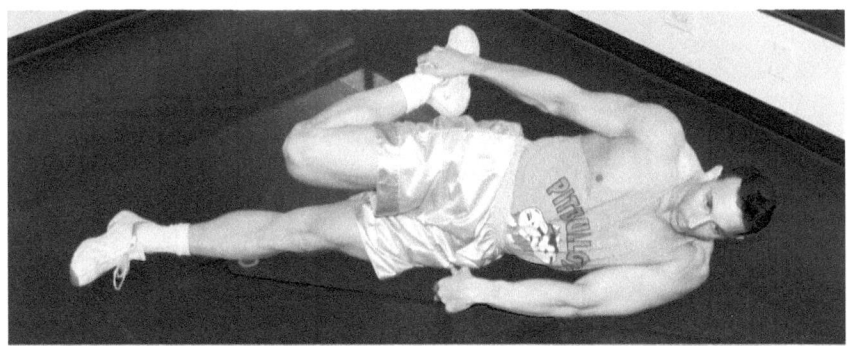

Lie on your side. Do a knee flexion toward your buttocks, grabbing your foot to complete the stretch.

Hamstring Stretches

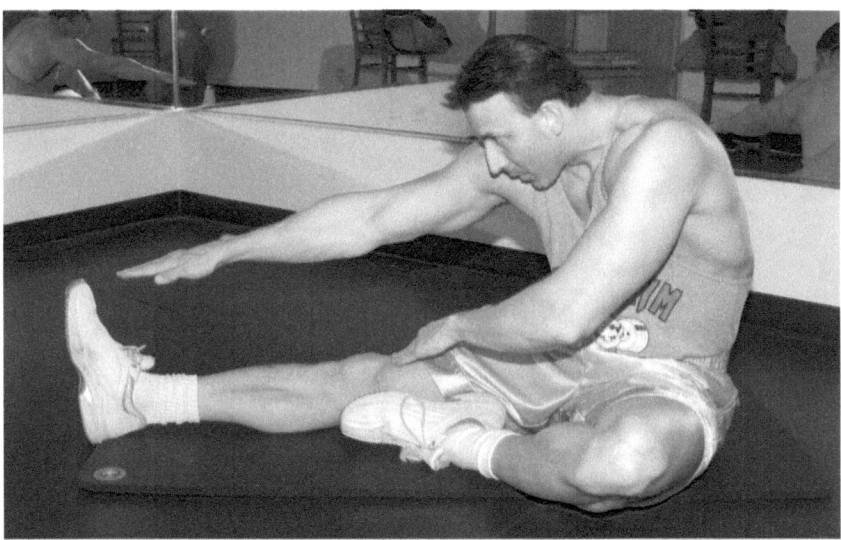

- Keeping one leg straight, tuck the opposite leg in an internal rotation and gradually reach down toward that foot.

Hamstring Stretch with a Towel

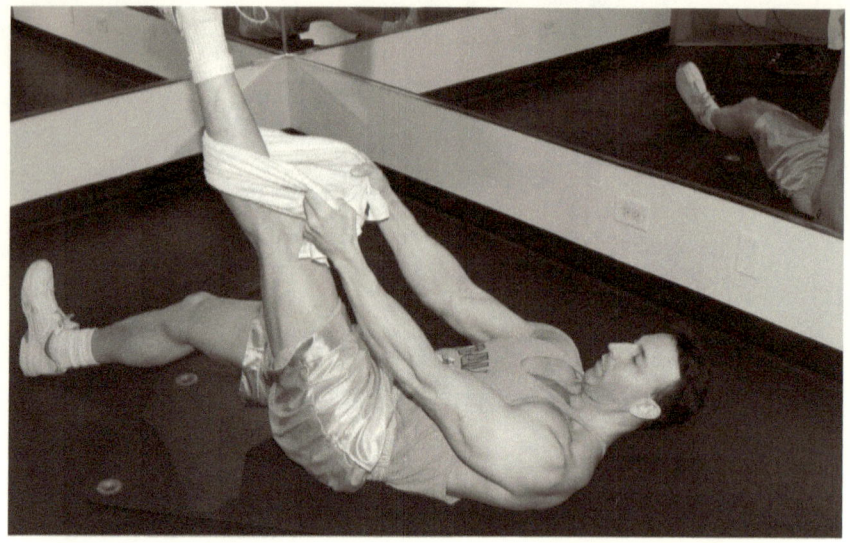

Place a towel around the calf of one leg and pull, keeping the leg straight and the opposite leg on the ground.

Hip Flexor Stretch

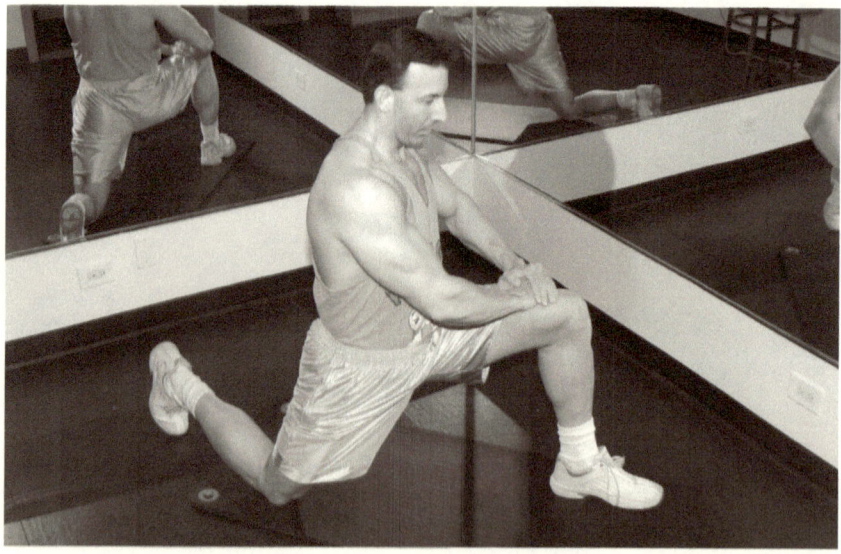

Kneel down on one foot, positioning the knee at 90 degrees and keeping the foot stationary. Slide your other foot as back far as possible, until the instep rests on the floor. Avoid rotating your spine.

Groin or Adductor Stretch (Butterflies)

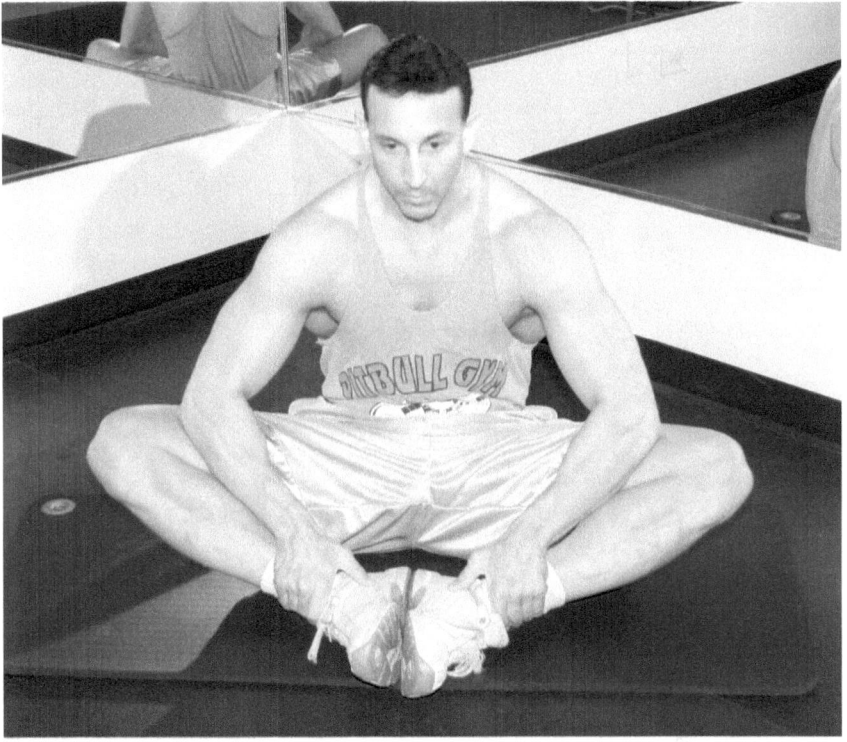

Sit with your back straight. Move both legs together in an internal rotation until the bottoms of both feet touch. Push your knees down with your elbows. Avoid applying too much pressure and pulling on the ankles. You can move your feet closer to or farther away from your body.

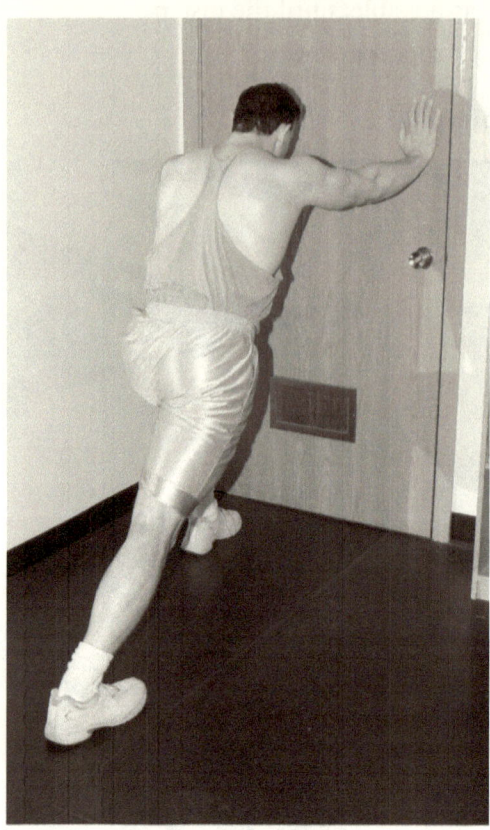

Gastrocnemius Stretch

Place your hands flat against a wall, and plant the back heel of the calf being stretched flat on the floor. Bend the front and stretch.

Soleus Stretch

Use a wall for support in this stretch. Place one foot behind the other. Keeping your knees straight, lean forward from your hips.

CHAPTER 7:
BODY PARTS, TARGETED MUSCLES, AND EXERCISES FOR BUILDING A NICE PHYSIQUE

In this chapter are some of the exercises I have done for every body part over the last twenty-five years.

The longer you train, the more important it is to use variations with different exercises. Always use different benches, bars, and other gym equipment. Change grips, handles, and angles often to hit the targeted muscles and surrounding muscle groups. For example, a flat bench press can work not only the pecs, it also can stimulate the triceps and front delts.

It's also important to change your routine and do different exercises for each muscle group so you can avoid hitting a plateau, as mentioned in Chapter 5. For example, when working your upper chest, do incline press one week, then do incline dumbbell flies the following week. Why? Muscle has memory. Muscle can grow only up to a point if you perform the same routine and exercises over and over. The muscles will adapt to the exercise, while other muscle fibers are neglected and need to be "shocked." Changing your workout routine, exercises, and frequency will change your body as you work different muscles and muscle fibers. It's OK to shock your muscles to stimulate growth, strength, and endurance.

Chest

Targeted Muscles: Pectorals, Anterior Deltoids, and Triceps

Pec Machine

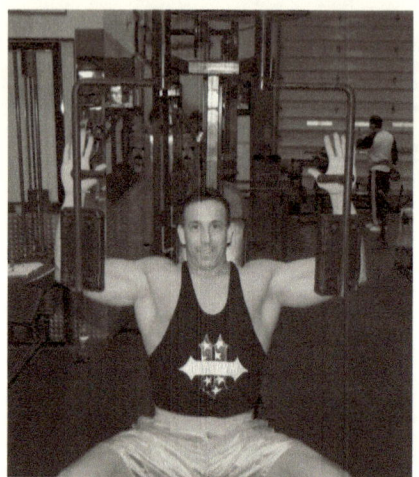 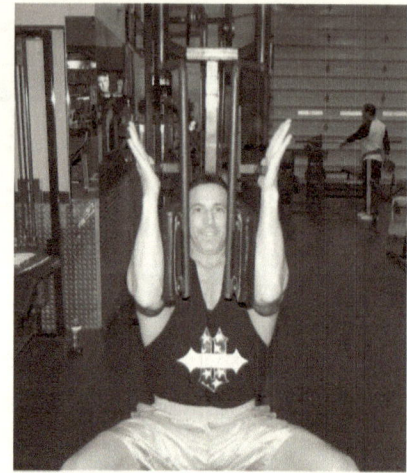

- Sit upright on the machine and adjust with your feet touching the ground.
- Keep palms open and stretch your chest as far as possible without strain.
- Inhale before your first repetition, then exhale while pulling the arm pads together, squeezing the chest muscles.
- At each repetition, when your arms meet together, control the movement on the way back to the starting position.
- Stretch the pectoral muscles by extending your arms as far back as they can go.

Incline Chest Press on the Smith Machine

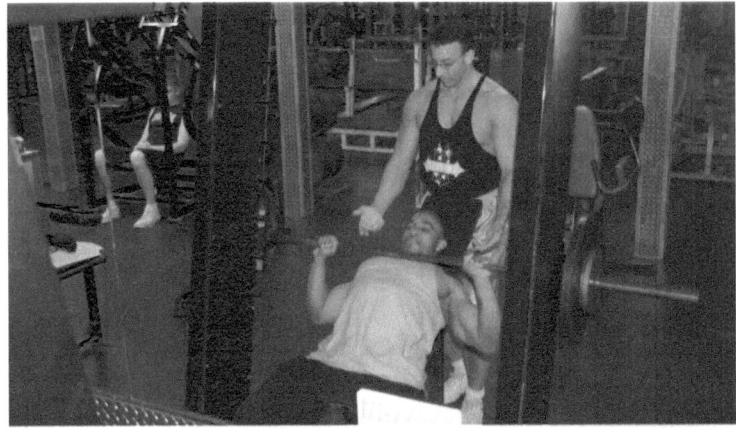

- Adjust the bench so that the bar is lined up with your upper chest.
- Align your hands with your little fingers covering the smooth mark on the bar.
- Lift and twist the bar to remove the clamps.
- Lower the weight while maintaining control.
- Extend the weight upward with a slight bend, but don't lock your arms.

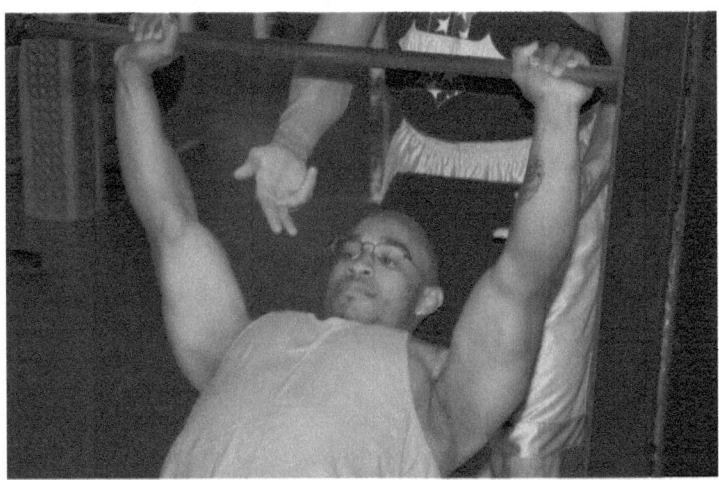

Incline Dumbbells Press

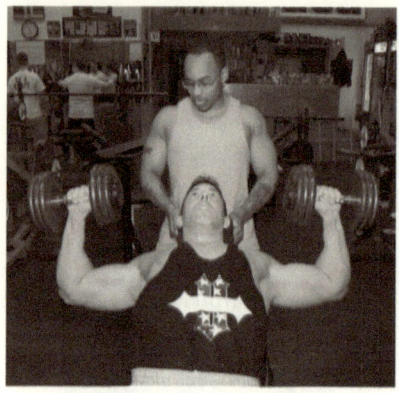 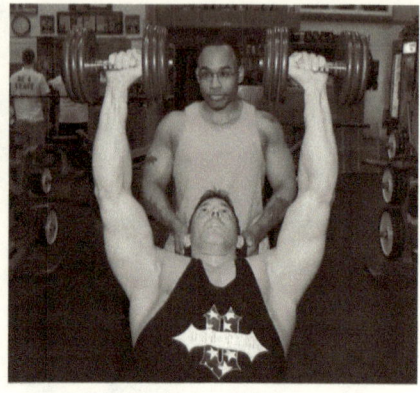

- Position the bench on a 20- to 45-degree incline.
- Hold the dumbbells lined up with your upper chest.
- Lower to the side.
- Extend your arms and squeeze your chest.

Flat Bench

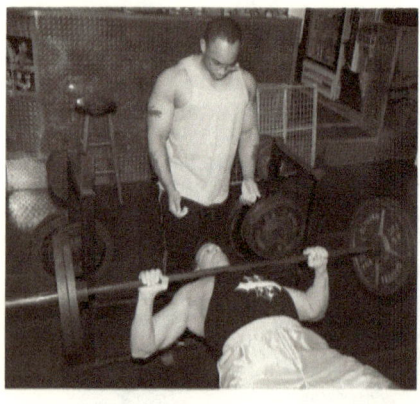 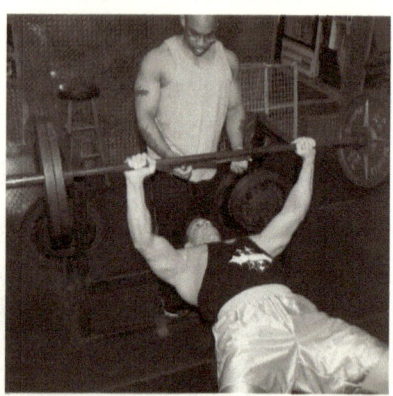

- Grip the barbell a fist-length-and-a-half outside your shoulder.
- Slowly lower the barbell toward your chest, lined up with your nipples.
- Inhale while lowering the barbell in a controlled motion.
- Exhale and push the weight upwards.

Flat Bench Dumbbell Press

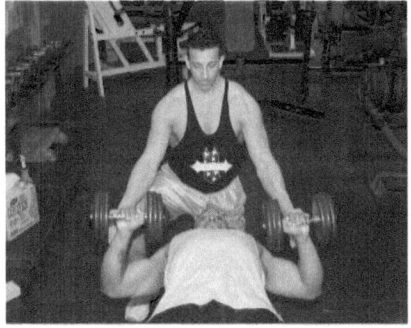 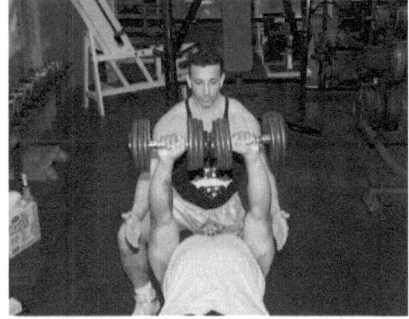

- Grip the dumbbells and hold them outside your shoulder.
- Line up the dumbbells mid-chest.
- Inhale and press the dumbbells directly upwards.
- Exhale and control the weight on the way down.

Decline Press

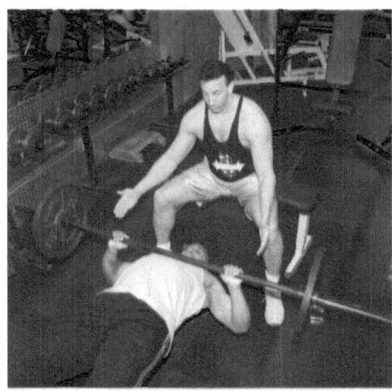 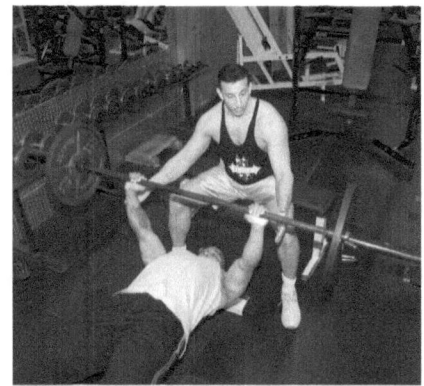

- Align your hands with your little fingers covering the smooth mark on the bar.
- Lower the bar underneath your pectoralis minor while inhaling.
- Push bar straight up and exhale.
- Lower the bar, controlling the movement.
- Extend your arms and squeeze your chest without locking your arms.

Shoulders

Targeted Muscles: Trapezius, Deltoids (Anterior, Medial, and Posterior), and Triceps

Shrugs

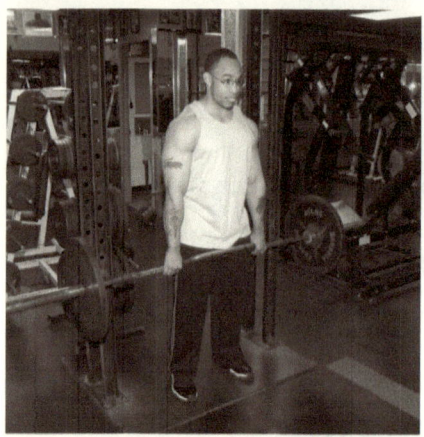 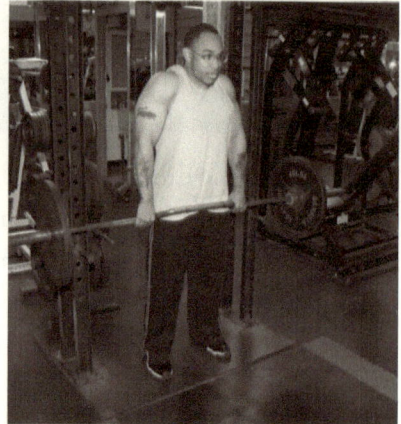

- Stand with your feet shoulder-width apart, knees slightly bent.
- Keep your back tight.
- Arms should be a fist apart from your thighs.
- Your arms should hang straight without bending throughout the movement.
- Lift the bar, keeping your arms straight and using your trapezius muscles to bring your shoulders up.

Seated Shoulder Press

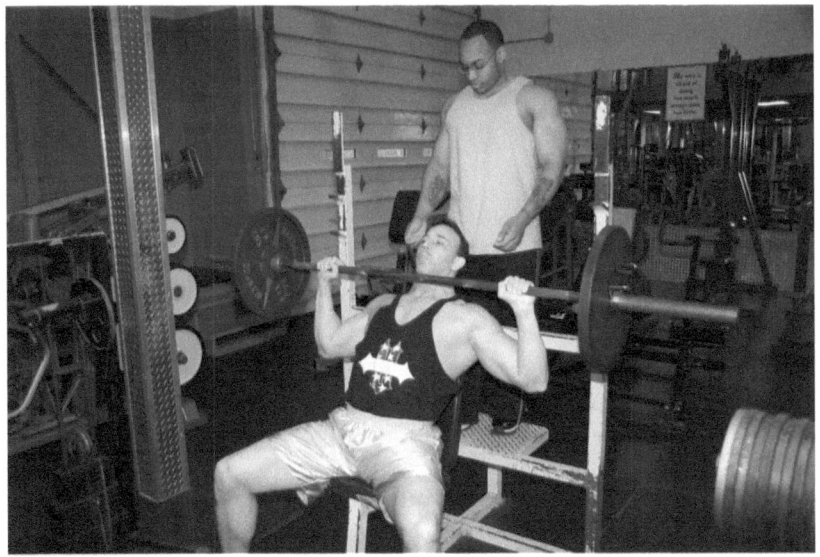

- Grip the bar with your little fingers lined up with the smooth marker on the bar.
- Lift and lower the bar to your chin, controlling the weight upward and downward.
- Press the bar overhead with arms slightly bent.
- Do not lock your arms.

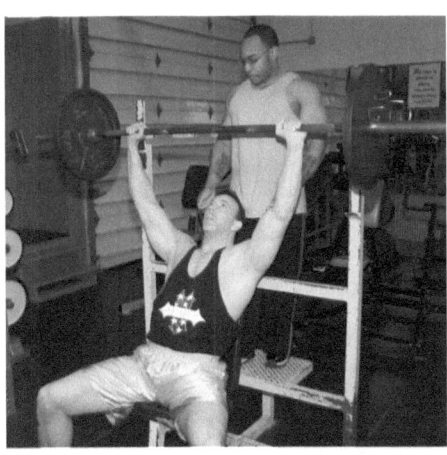

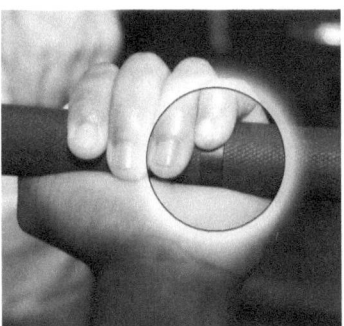

Seated Dumbbell Press

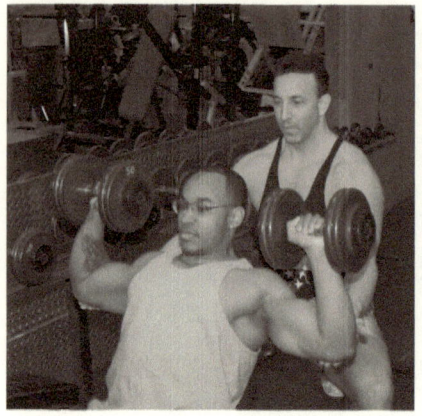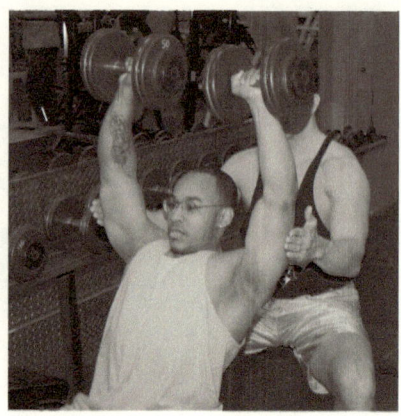

- Stabilize in a seated posture.
- Start with the dumbbells outside your shoulders.
- Inhale, then exhale while pressing the dumbbells overhead.
- Lower the dumbbells, controlling the movement.

Lateral Raises

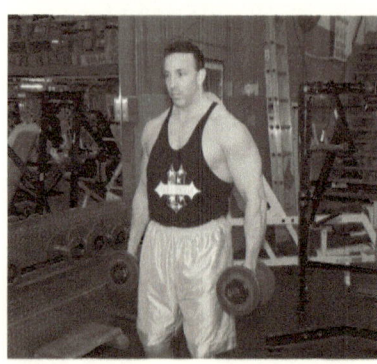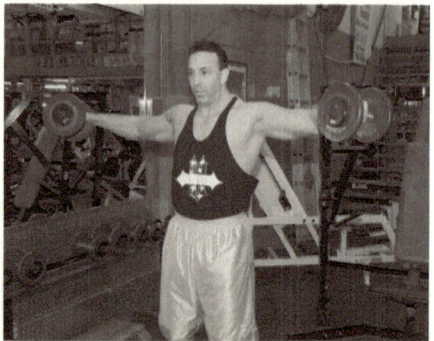

- Stand with your feet shoulder-width apart, knees slightly bent.
- Keep your body upright and core-tight.
- Hold the dumbbells at your sides.
- Keeping your elbows slightly bent, raise your arms until they are parallel with the ground.
- Lower the dumbbells back to the starting position, controlling the movement.

Prone Dumbbell Rear Pull, Working the Rear Deltoids

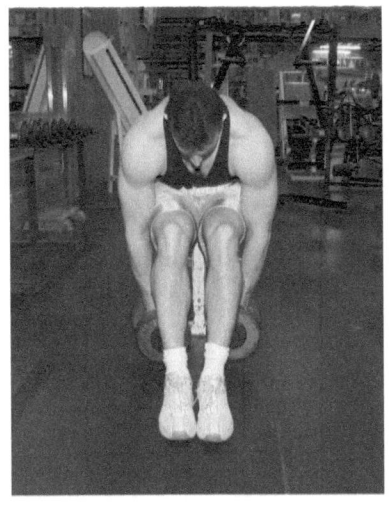 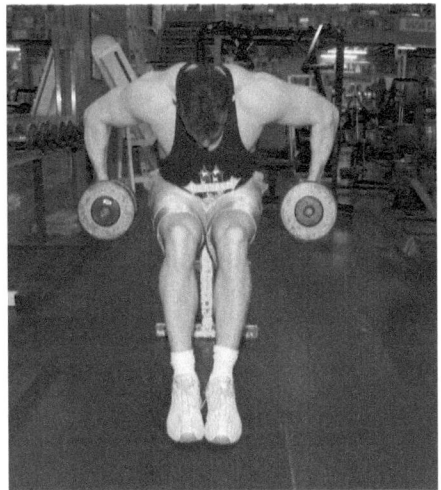

- Sit on the edge of a flat bench with your legs extended and feet flat.
- Bend your upper torso over your legs.
- Grip the dumbbells underneath your legs.
- Lift the dumbbells, retracting your shoulder blades and leading with your elbows.
- Keep your head and neck aligned with your spine.

BACK

TARGETED MUSCLES: LATISSIMUS DORSI, TERES MAJOR, RHOMBOIDS, BICEPS, POSTERIOR DELTOIDS, AND LEVATOR SCAPULAE

Lat Pull-Down

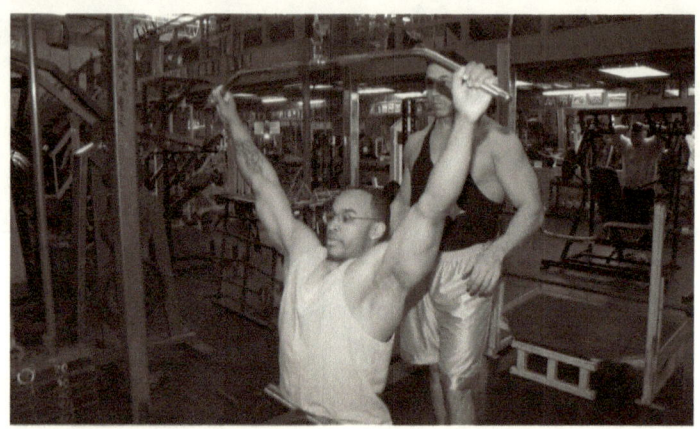

- Use a wide grip on the bar.
- Stabilize your body in a seated position.
- Lean back approximately 75 degrees.
- Pull the bar to your upper chest.
- Inhale before the first rep, and exhale while pulling down.
- Control the bar on the way to the up position.

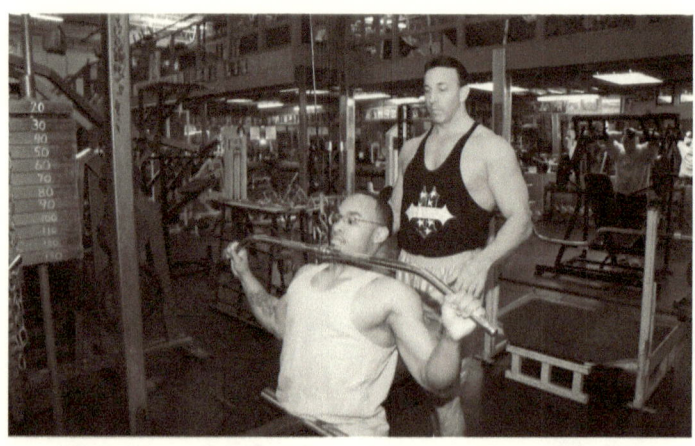

Seated Cable Row

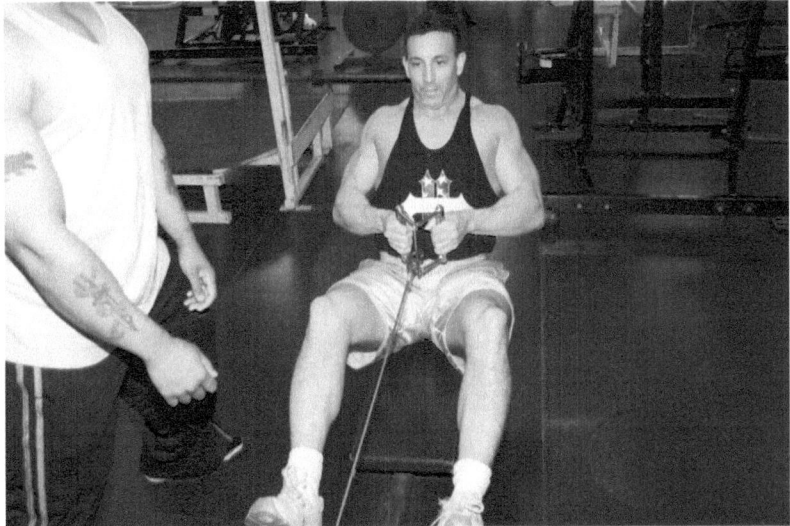

- Stabilize your lower body, keeping your knees slightly bent.
- Hold your chest and stabilize your spine and pelvis.
- Inhale while reaching for the cable.
- Pull the handles toward your body at the lower chest, above the abdominals.
- Retract your shoulders and squeeze your back.
- Extend your arms and stretch your back when returning to the starting position.

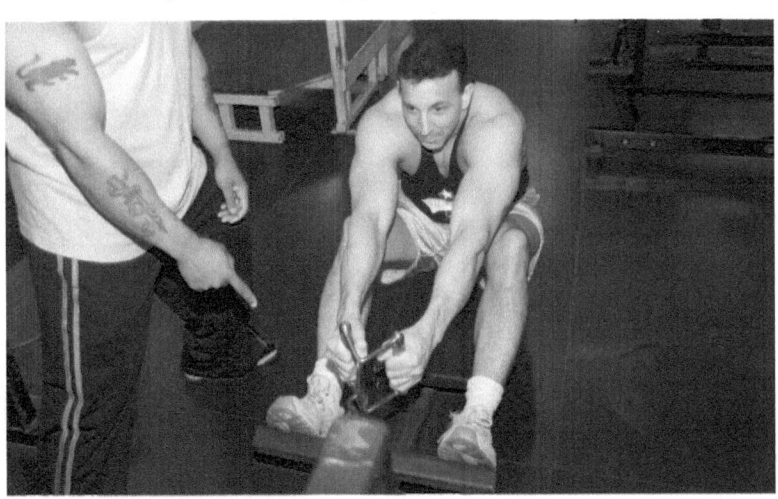

Bent-Over Barbell Rows with Straight Bar (Prone and Supinated Grip)

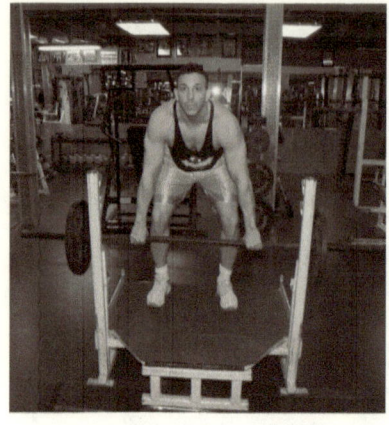 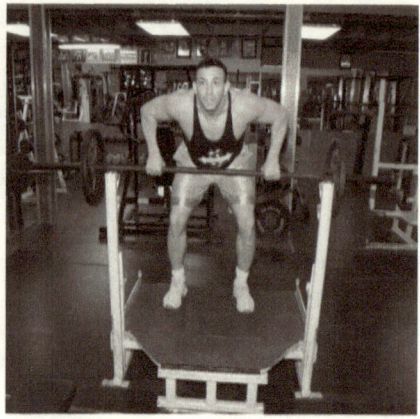

- Position your feet shoulder-width apart.
- Bend at the waist, keeping your knees slightly bent.
- Keep your back and head straight, looking straight ahead.
- Raise the bar toward your body.
- Focus on working your back, not your arms.

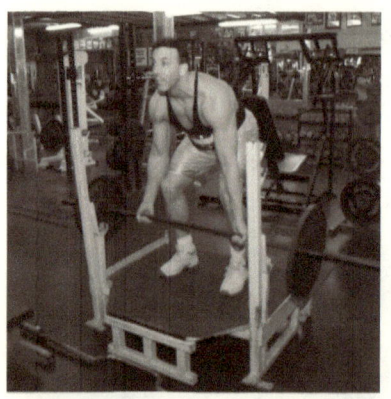 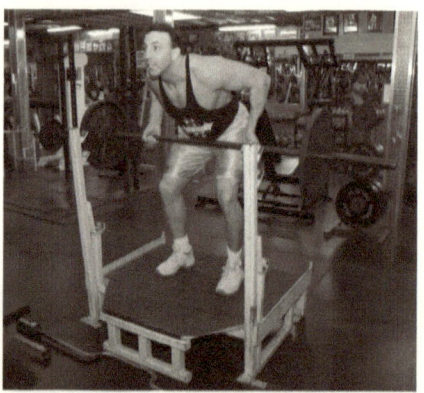

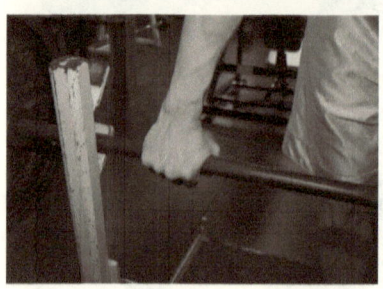 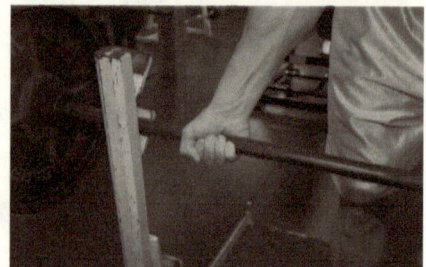

Pull-Ups

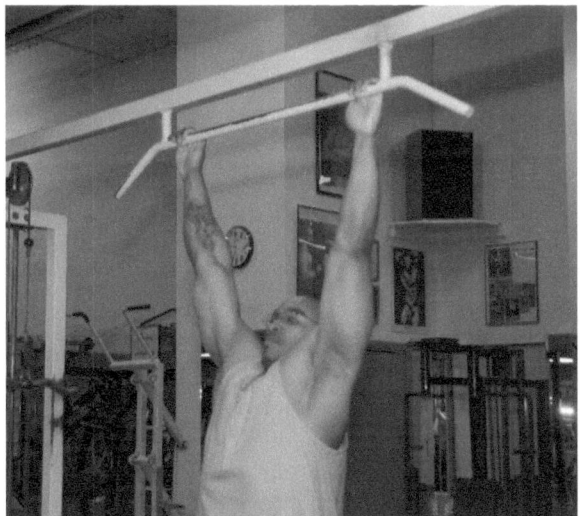

- Grip the chin-up bar with an overhand grip, placing your hands as far apart as possible.
- Hang from the bar with your arms extended.
- Pull up towards the bar until your upper chest touches the bar.
- Hold and squeeze for 1 second, then lower to the starting position.

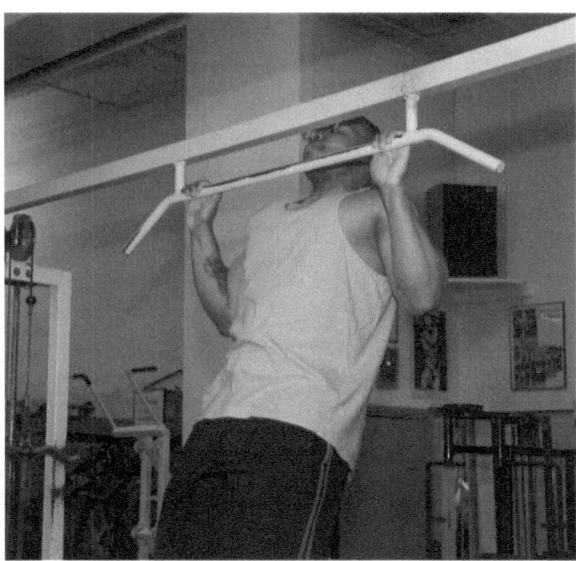

Dead Lifts

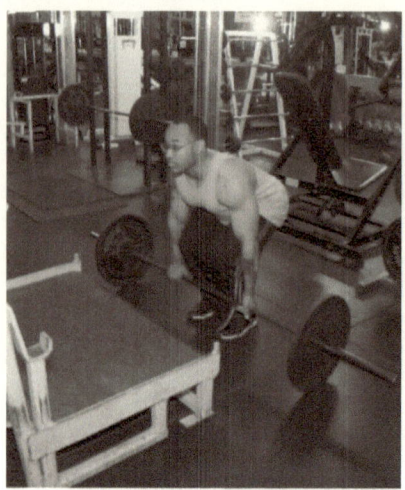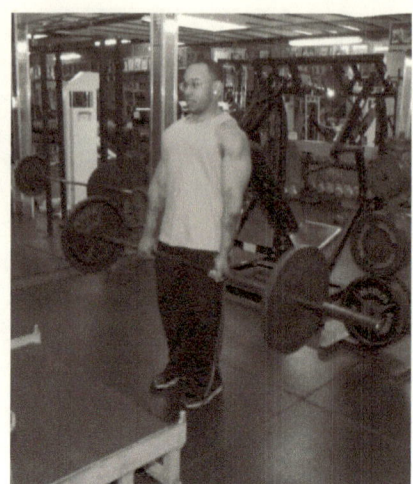

- Grip the bar in front using an overhand grip with one hand and an underhand grip with the other hand.
- Your hands should be in a medium-wide grip just outside shoulder width.
- Bend your knees and lean forward while keeping your back straight. Avoid curving your back.
- Drive with your legs to a standing position.
- Move your chest out and your shoulders back.
- To lower the weight back down to the floor, bend your knees and lean forward from the waist.

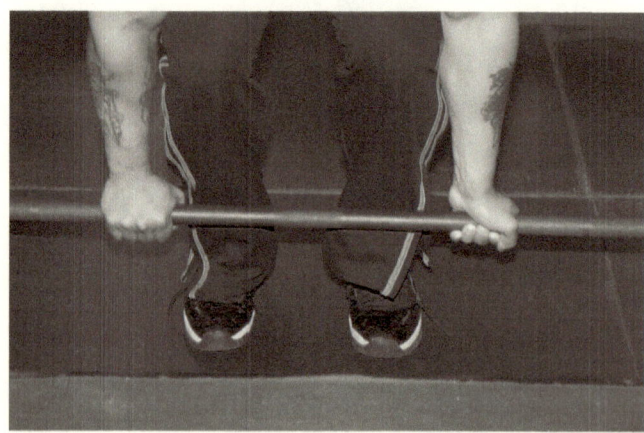

Hyperextensions

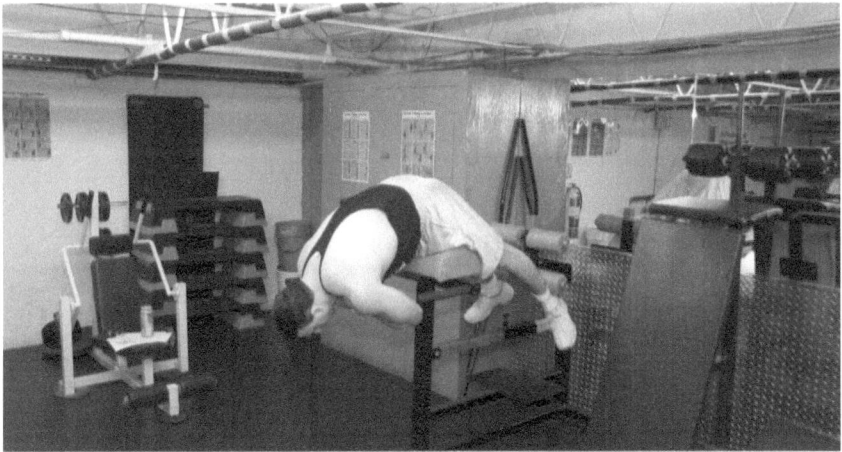

- Lie in a prone position and adjust the hyperextension board.
- Place your heels firmly under the foot support.
- Make sure your hip joint is above the pad and your lower torso is stabilized.
- Keep your arms crossed in front of your chest.
- Lower your body forward, stretching your back and hamstrings.
- Lift your body up as far as you can go, squeezing your lower back and gluteus maximus.

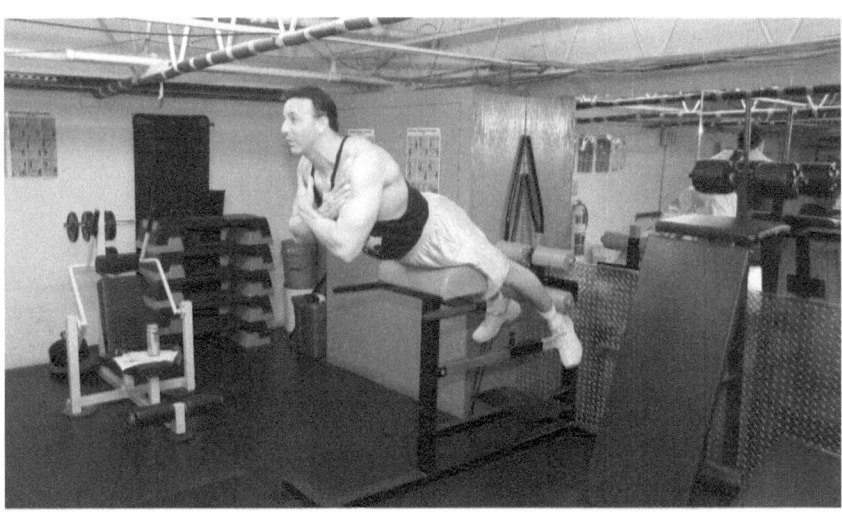

BICEPS

TARGET MUSCLES: BICEPS BRACHII, BRACHIALIS, AND BRACHIORADIALIS

Standing Biceps Curl with Straight Bar

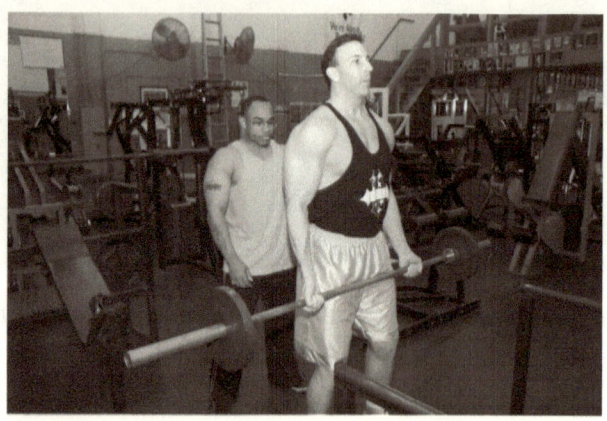

- Position your feet shoulder-width apart, keeping your core tight.
- Keep your elbows at your sides.
- Grip the bar with a supinated hand grip.
- Curl the bar, keeping your elbows in and your back tight.
- Squeeze your biceps as you lift.
- Return to the starting position, keeping the movement controlled.

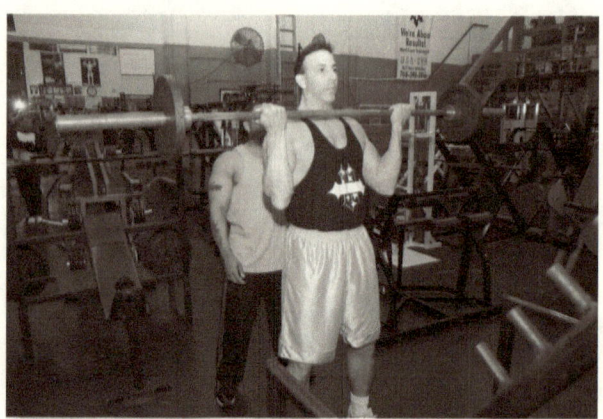

Single-Arm Isolation Curls (Peak Builders)

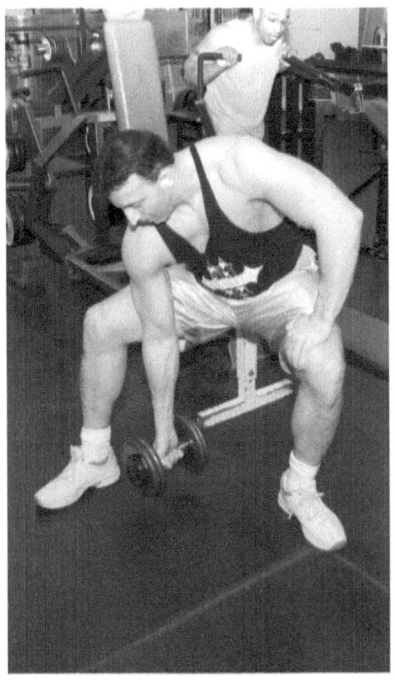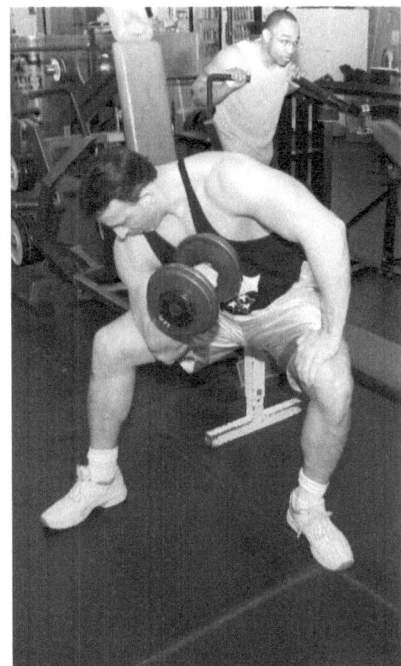

- Sit on the edge of a flat bench with your legs in an L-shape.
- Place your elbow against your thigh.
- Hold the dumbbell with a supinated grip.
- Curl your arm while twisting your wrist in an external rotation.
- Keep your body erect.

Overhead Cable Curls

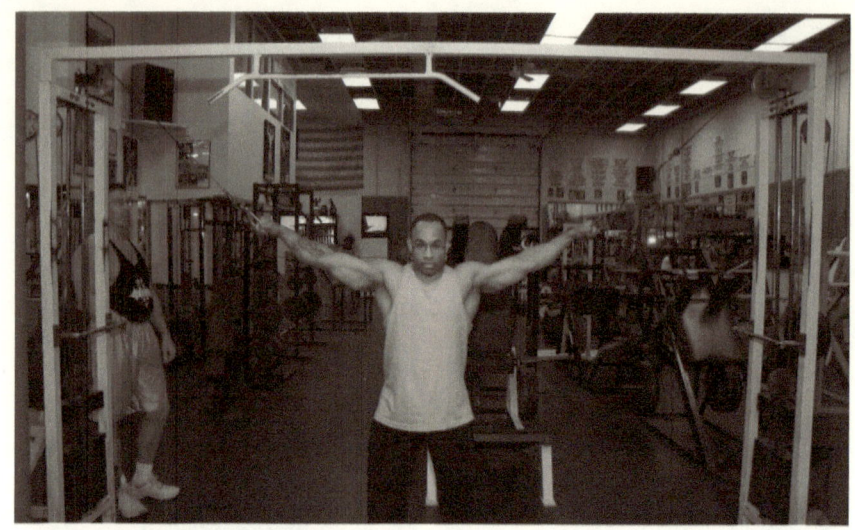

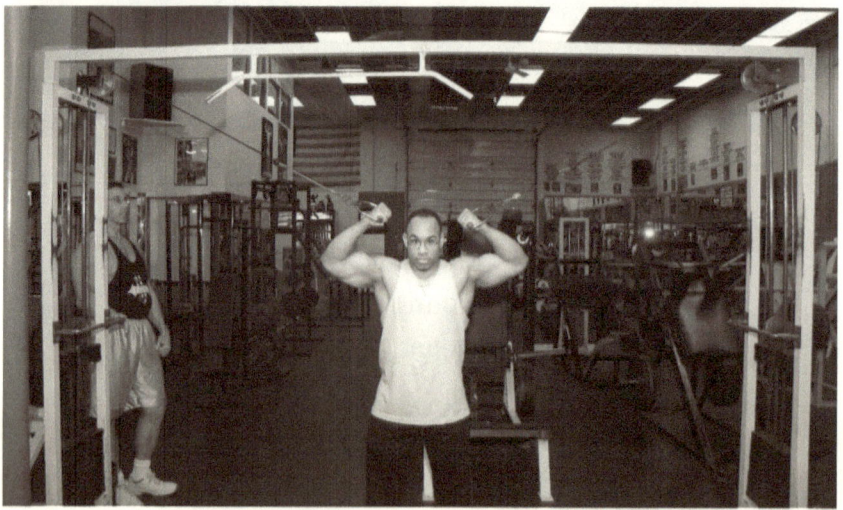

- Stand between two pulleys with your feet shoulder-width apart.
- Grip the attachments with your palms facing away from your body.
- Position your arms at a 35-degree angle.
- Twist your wrists inward while pulling the attachments toward your head.
- Squeeze your biceps while keeping your back straight.
- Return your arms to the starting position, keeping the movement controlled.

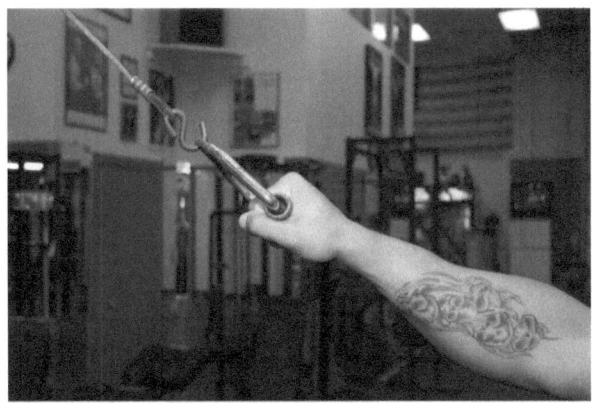

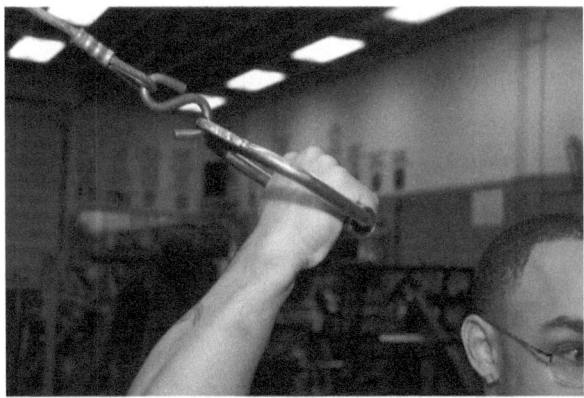

Reverse Curls with Hands in a Prone Grip Using the E-Z Bar

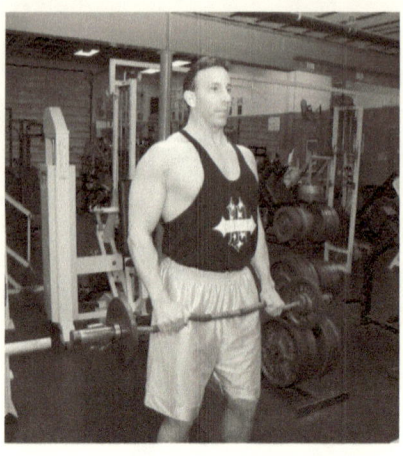 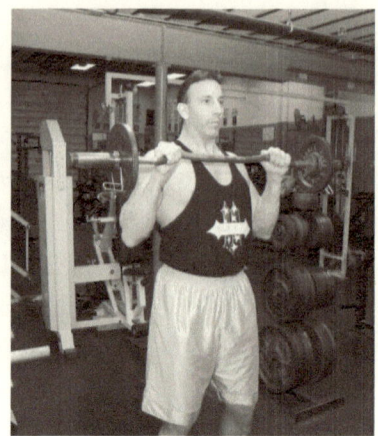

The E-Z bar is a bent and curved bar especially designed for curling.

- Position your feet shoulder-width apart,
  keeping your core tight.
- Keep your elbows at your sides, as far back as possible.
- Curl the bar toward your chest.

TRICEPS

TARGET MUSCLES: TRICEPS BRACHII—MEDIAL HEAD, LATERAL HEAD, AND LONG HEAD

When working triceps, place your thumbs on the same side as the other fingers when gripping. Don't wrap thumbs around the bar or machine.

Standing Triceps Push-Downs with Rope

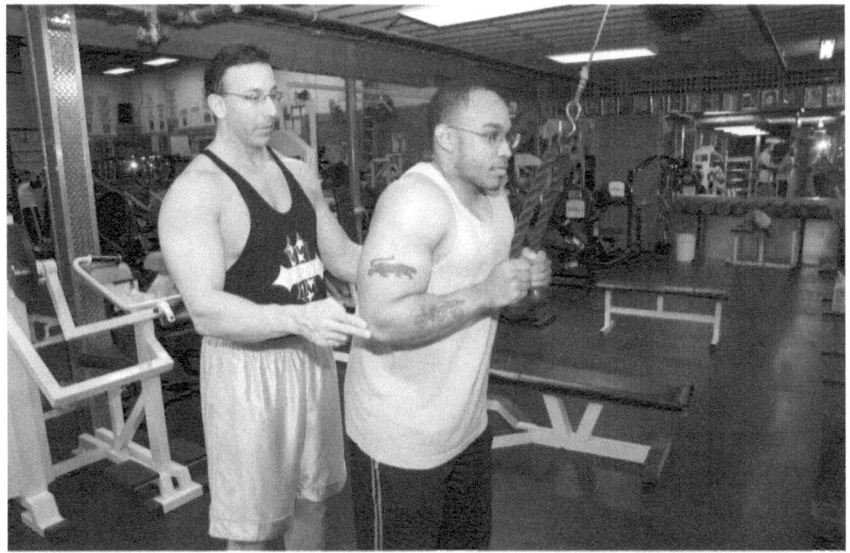

- Position your feet shoulder-width apart.
- Bend your knees slightly, keeping your core tight.
- Keep your elbows at your sides.
- Position the rope at mid-chest.
- Inhale and exhale, pushing the rope down and out.

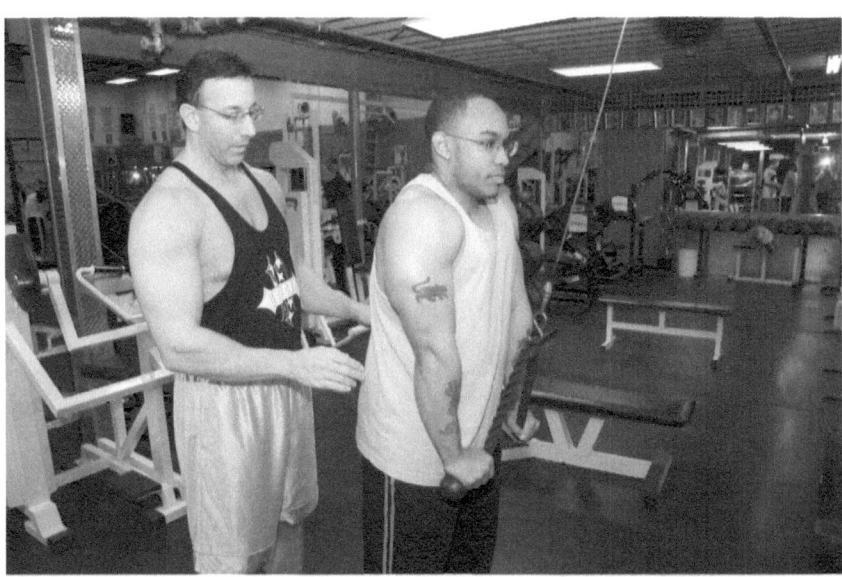

Lying Triceps Extension (Skull Crushers) Using the E-Z Bar

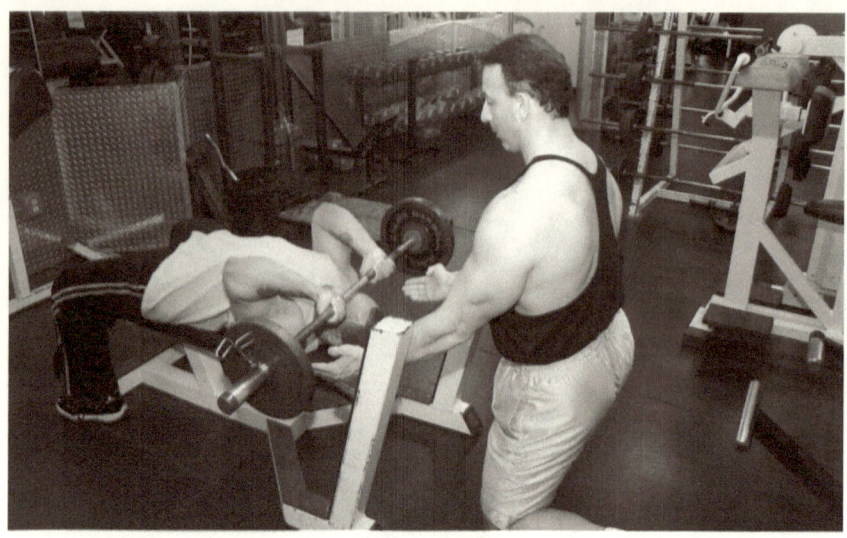

- Lie in a supine position on a flat bench.
- Grasp the E-Z bar on the inner grip of the bar.
- Keep your elbows in and stabilized above the shoulder joint.
- Bend your elbows and lower the bar to two inches above your forehead. Maintain control of the bar.
- Exhale and extend your elbows while stabilizing your shoulders.

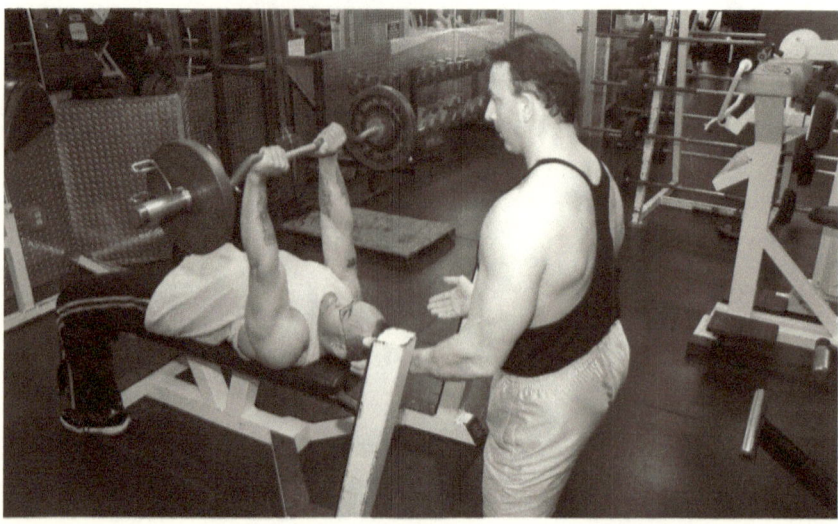

Overhead Triceps Extensions

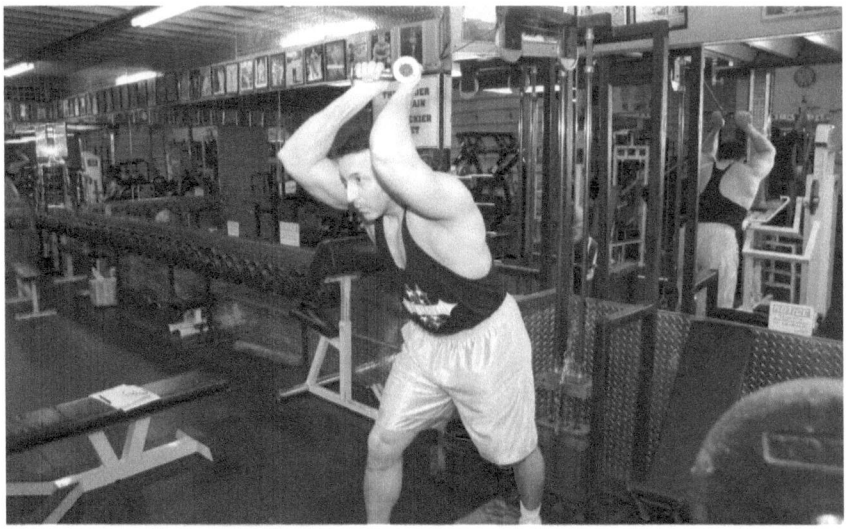

- Stand with your back to the weights.
- Grip the attachment with your hands facing each other.
- Keep your elbows in and bend at the waist
  until your arms are at a 90-degree angle.
- Push the attachment forward until
  your arms are fully extended.
- Control to the starting position, stretching the triceps.

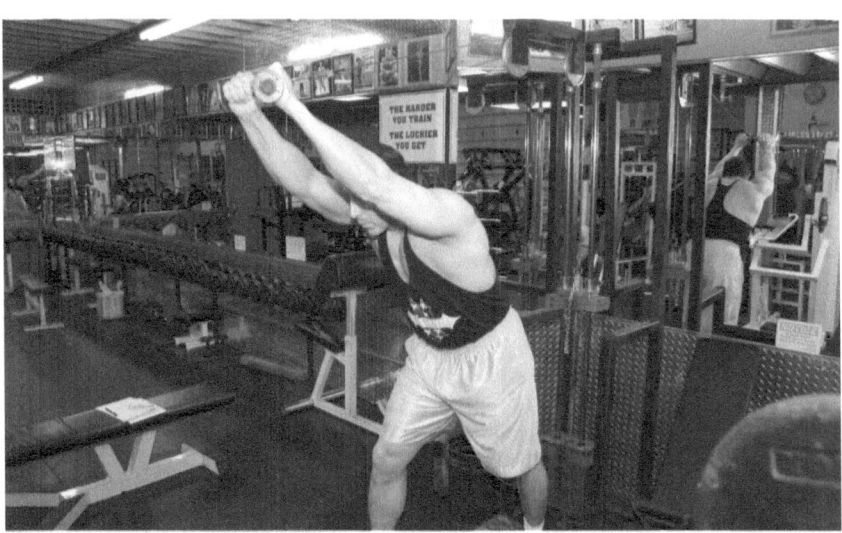

Triceps Push-Downs with Machine

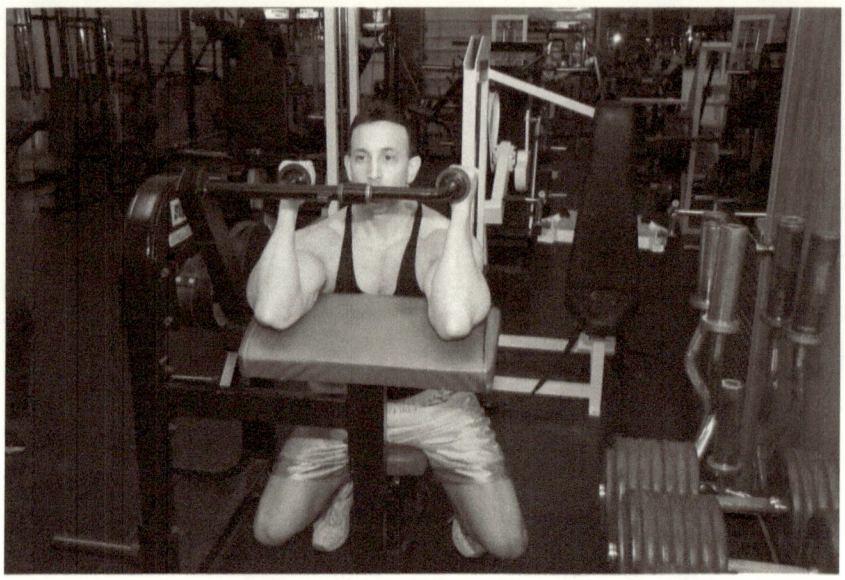

- Grip the handles.
- Push the weight down while keeping your body stabilized.
- Control the weight on the return to the starting position.

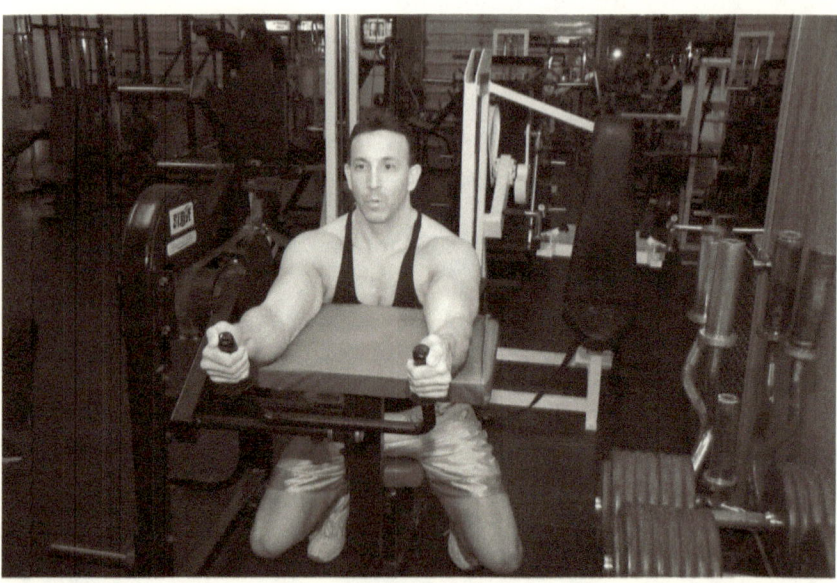

Dips

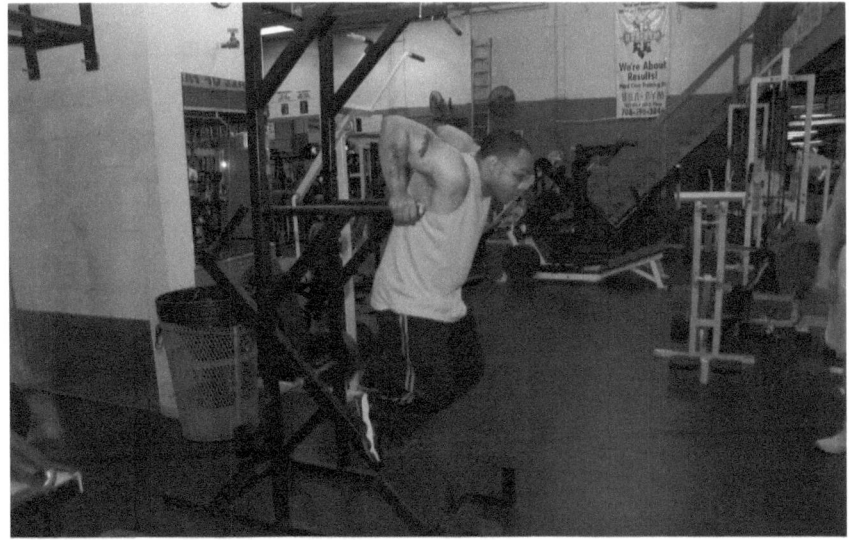

- Hold the bars with your arms locked.
- Keep your body upright.
- Lower your body between the bars as far down as you can without going too deep.
- Push up and lock your arms.

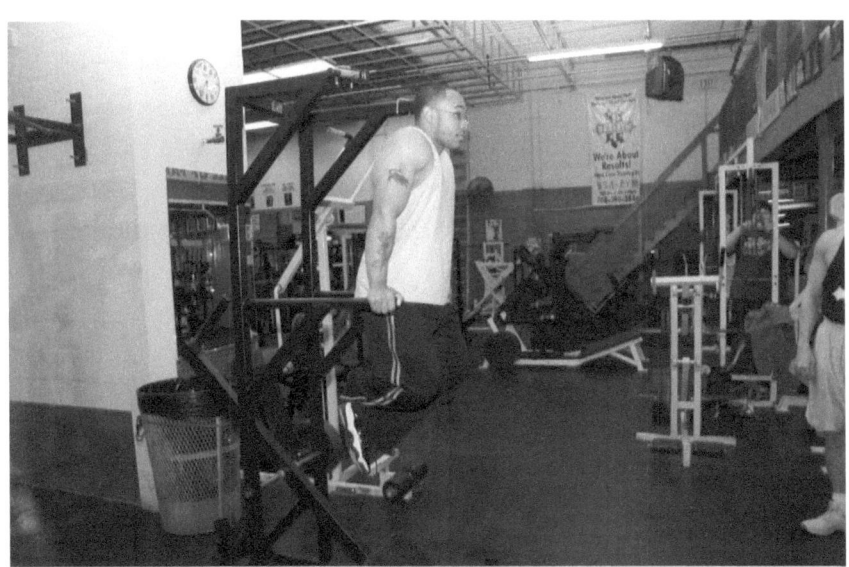

LEGS

TARGET MUSCLES: QUADRICEPS, ILIOPSOAS, GLUTEUS MAXIMUS, HAMSTRINGS, TIBIALIS ANTERIOR, GASTROCNEMIUS, SOLEUS, AND PERONEALS

Leg Extensions

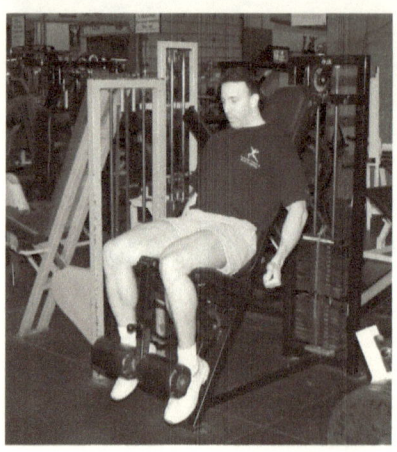 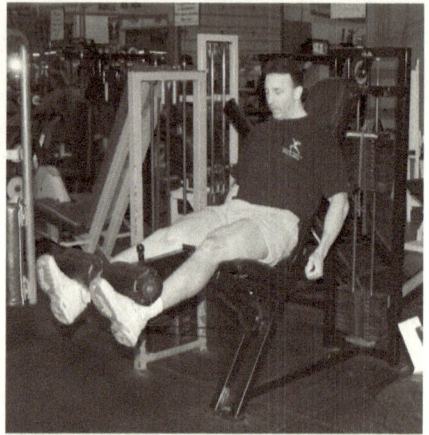

- Sit upright on the leg-extension machine.
- Align feet and knees shoulder-width apart.
- Hold the handgrips on the side of the machine and remain firmly planted in the seated position.
- Place your feet underneath the pads and extend your legs to maximum length.
- Control the weight on the return to the starting position.

Squats

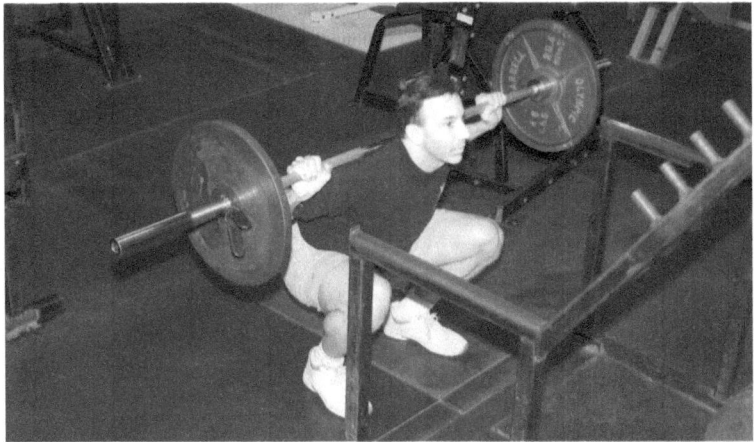

- Position your body under the squat rack. The bar should rest on your shoulders and upper traps.
- Place your feet shoulder-width apart.
- Lift the bar off the rack and step back in a standing position.
- Lower your body by bending your knees until your thighs are lower than parallel to your knees.
- Drive your legs back to the starting position.
- Monitor the weight and the length of the downward position if you have knee problems.

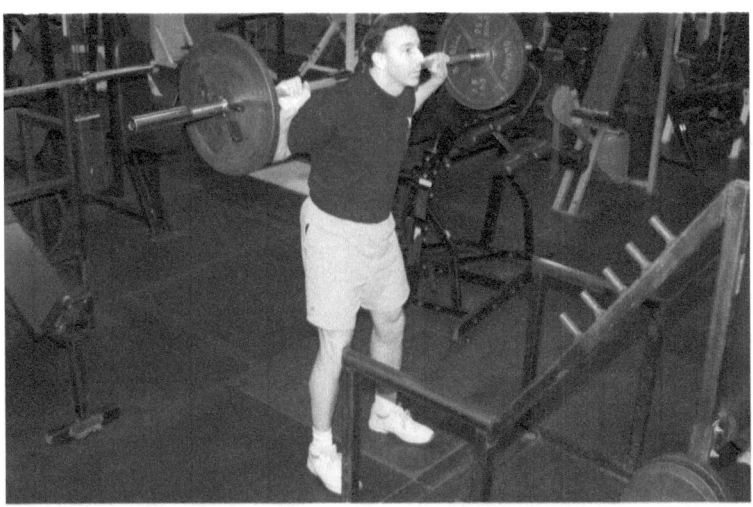

Leg Press

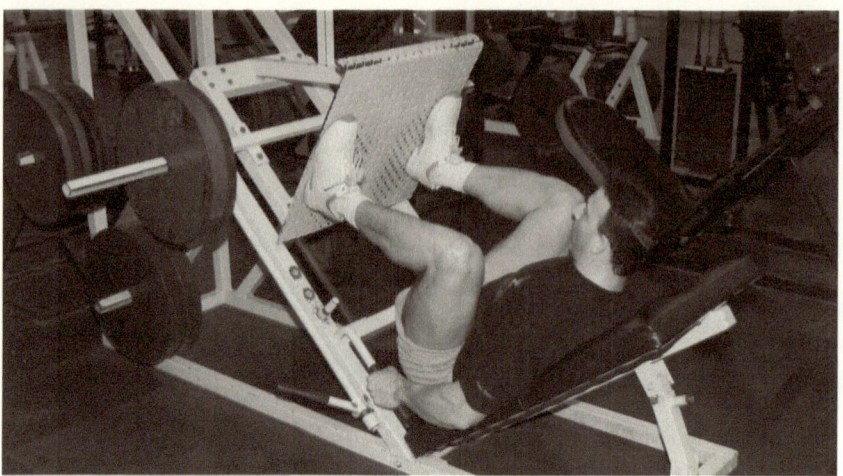

- Place both feet against the end of the plate on the leg-press machine.
- Hold the side handgrips on the machine.
- Bring the weight down to your body in a controlled manner.
- Push the weight back, keeping your knees slightly bent. Don't lock them.
- Return the weight to the starting position.

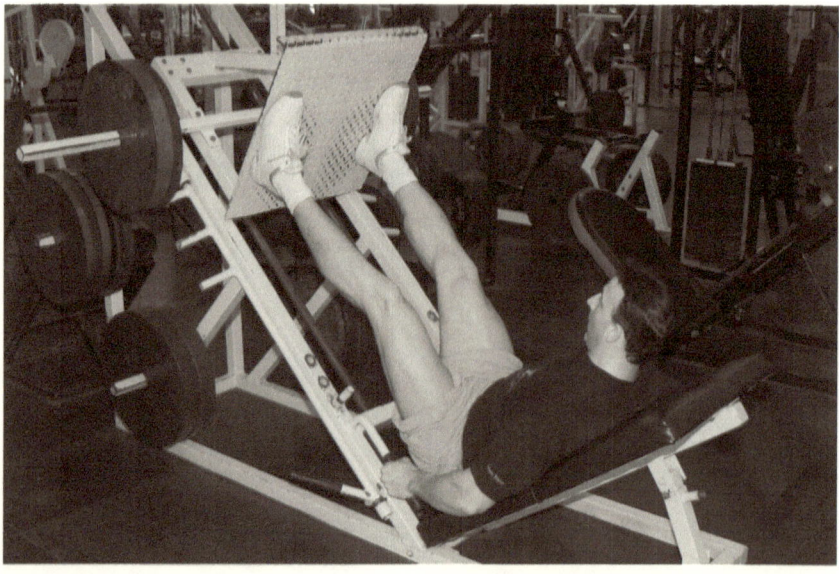

Lunges

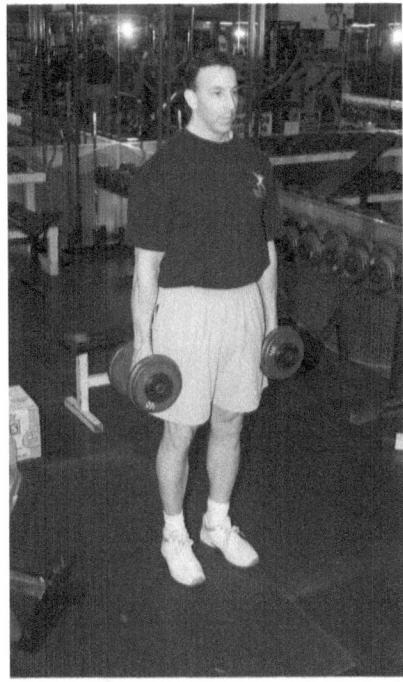 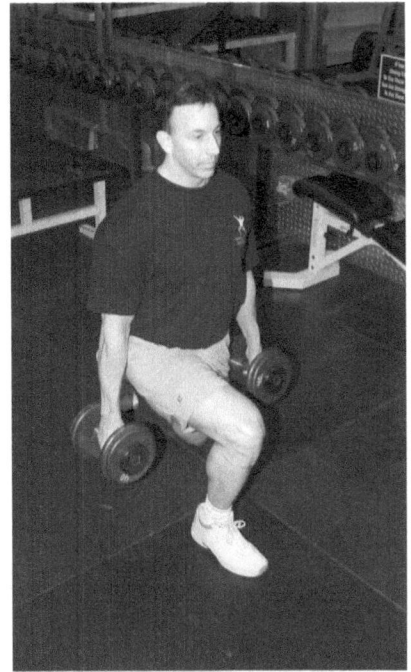

- Start with your feet together, holding the
  dumbbells at your sides with arms extended.
- Take a long step forward. Do not lunge
  your front knee past your toes.
- Lower your back knee straight down until it is an inch away
  from the floor. Keep your back straight and arms hanging.
- Push back up to the original standing position and repeat.

Hamstring Curls in a Prone Position

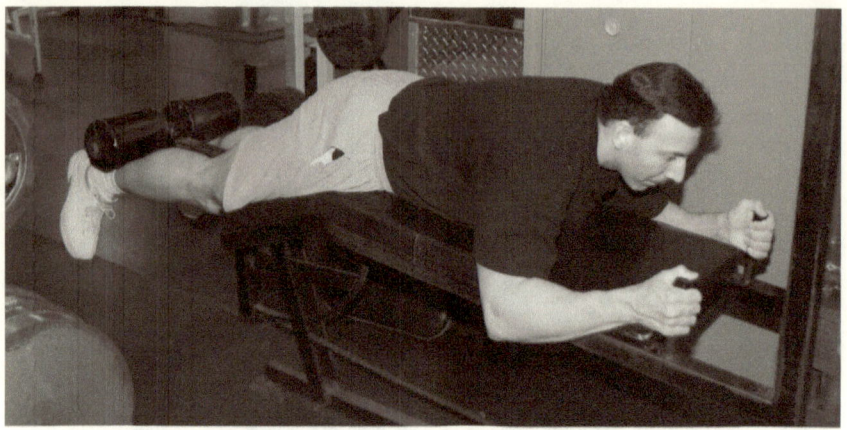

- Lying on your stomach, place your feet just under the bench bar. Keep your knees slightly bent.
- Curl the weight with your feet toward your buttocks.
- Return the weight to the starting position.

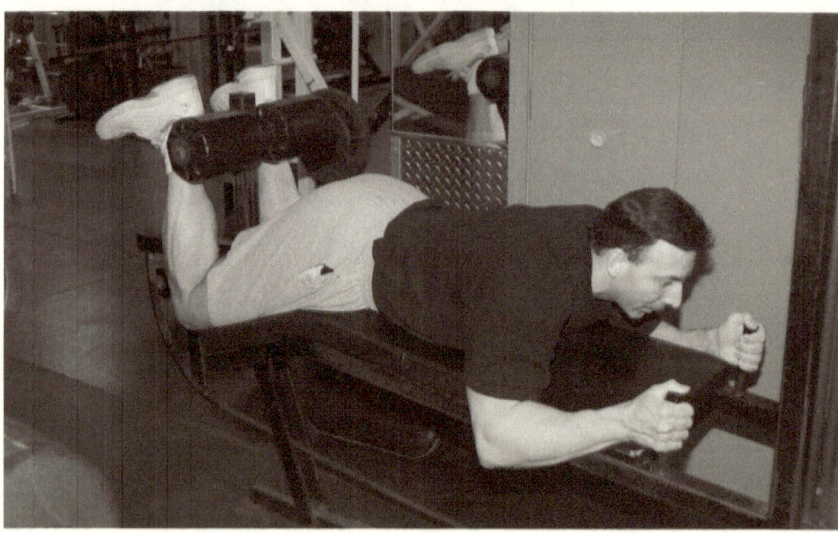

Hip Abductors/Adductors Using the Abductor/Adductor Machine

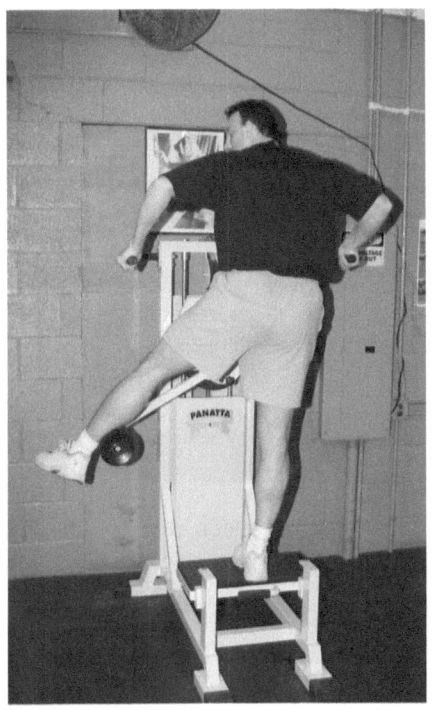 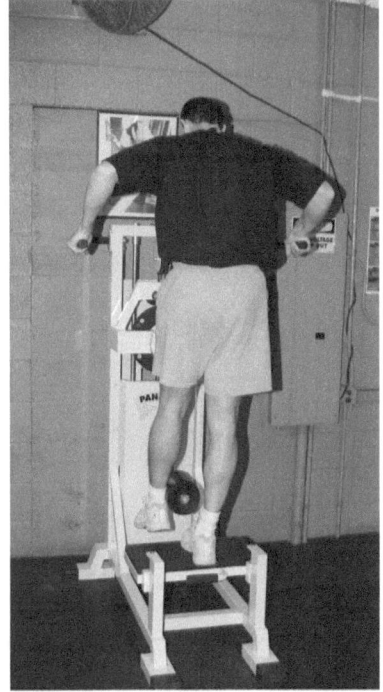

"Abduction" means to move the leg *away from* the midpoint of the body. "Adduction" means to move the leg *toward* the midpoint of the body.

- Place your ankle against the pad on the abductor/adductor machine.
- Keep your back foot straight on the middle of the platform.
- Stabilize your body.
- Engage the abductor or adductor movement in a controlled fashion.

Calf Raises

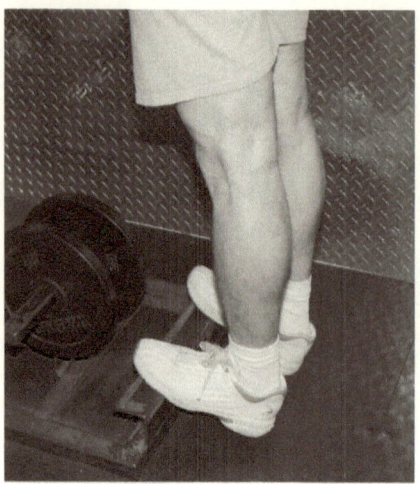 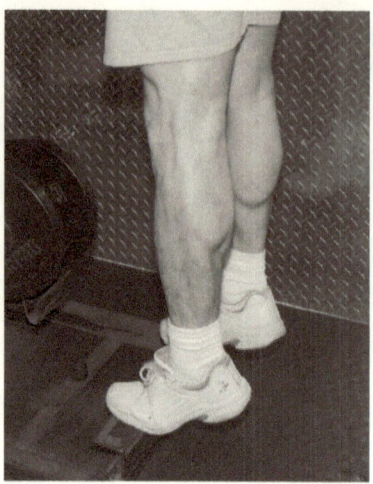

- Place your shoulders underneath the calf machine.
- Position your feet shoulder-width apart.
- Rest the balls of your feet on the platform.
- Dip your heels as far down as they can go on the platform.
- Push the weight up using the balls of your feet.
- Extend your feet as far as possible.
- Return the weight slowly to the starting position.

ABDOMINALS

Having strong core or abdominal muscles is key to maintaining good overall fitness and athleticism. A strong core can help prevent lower back pain and injuries as well as strength imbalance. Abdominal muscles can be worked *every day*.

Crunches

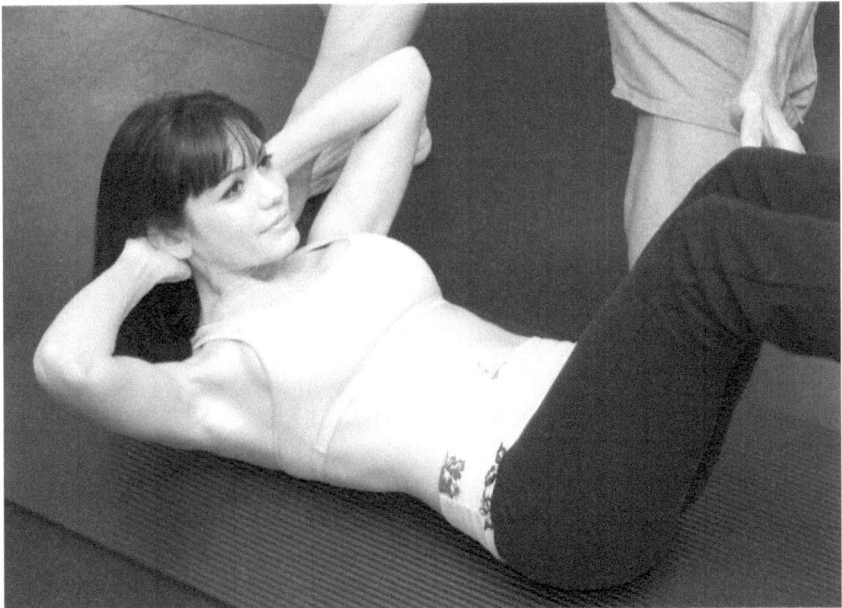

- Lie flat on your back.
- Place your fingertips behind your head for support without putting pressure on the head and neck.
- Do not force resistance on the head.
- Lift your knees, keeping hips flexed at 90 degrees.
- Keep your shoulder blades off the floor.
- Tuck your chin to your chest.
- Sit up, lifting your upper body as high as possible.
- Slowly return your upper body to the starting position, rolling the back.

Crunches with Feet in Butterfly Position

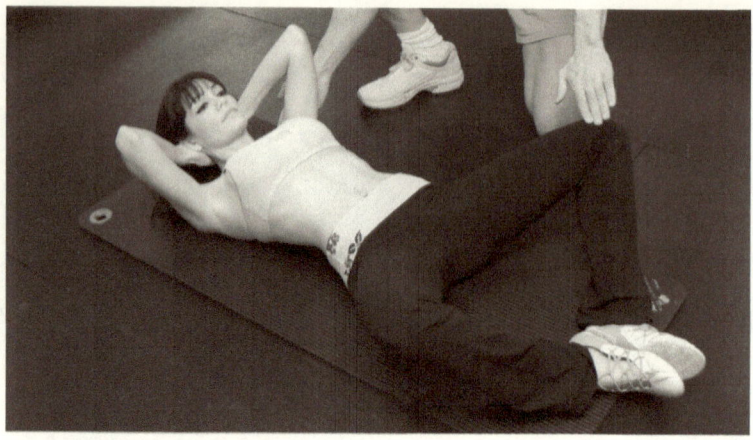

- Lie flat on your back.
- Place your fingertips behind your head for support without putting pressure on the head and neck.
- Do not force resistance on the head.
- Bend your knees and put the bottoms of your feet together in the butterfly position.
- Keep your shoulder blades off the floor.
- Tuck your chin to your chest.
- Sit up, lifting your upper body as high as possible.
- Slowly return your upper body to the starting position, rolling the back.

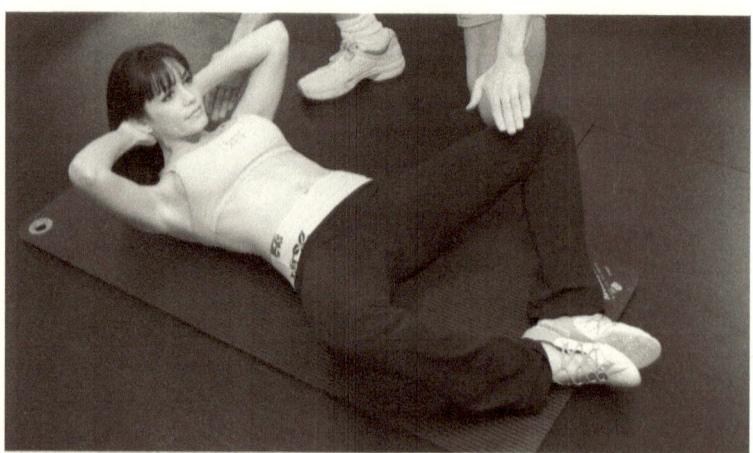

Legs Up at 90-degree Reach

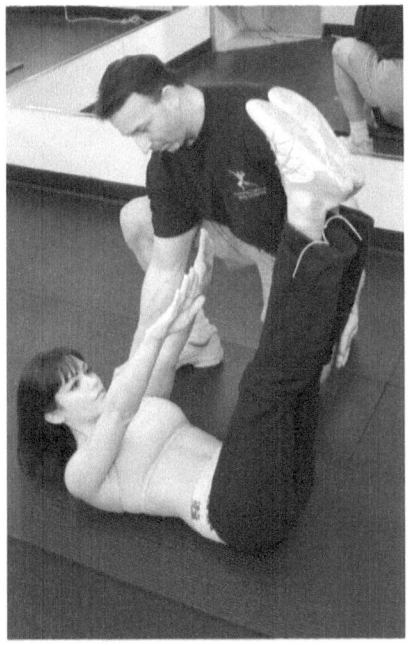 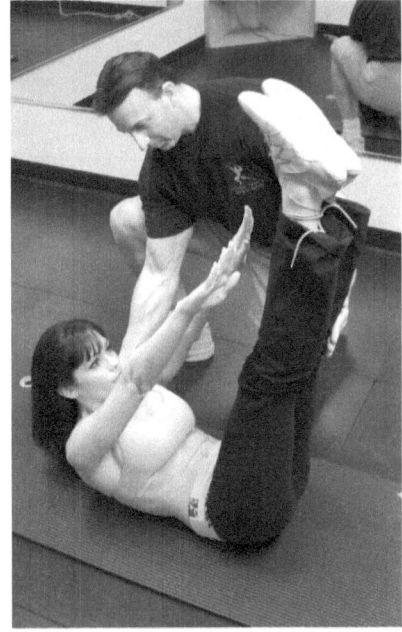

- Position your legs straight upward, perpendicular to the floor.
- Keep your knees straight and hips at 90 degrees.
- Straighten your arms and reach up toward your feet, contracting your abs.

Side Bends with Knees Bent

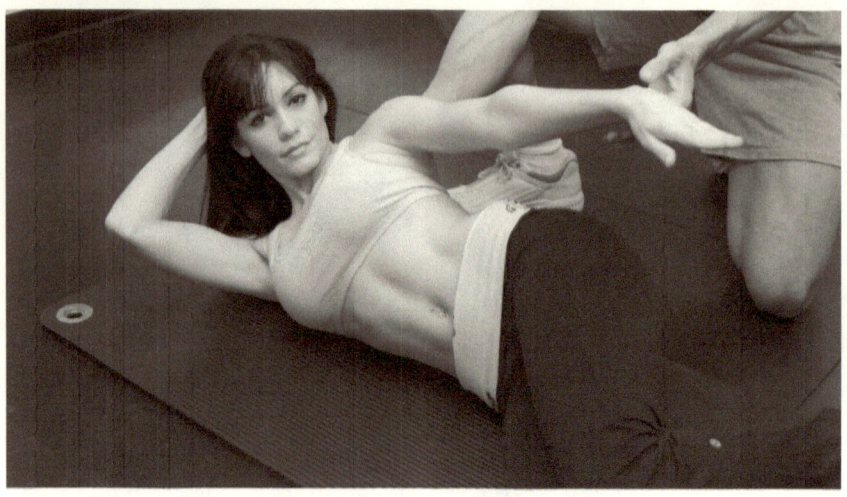

- Lie on your side with your knees bent.
- Align your feet with your hips.
- Straighten your arm along the side of your body.
- Contract the obliques as far as they can go.

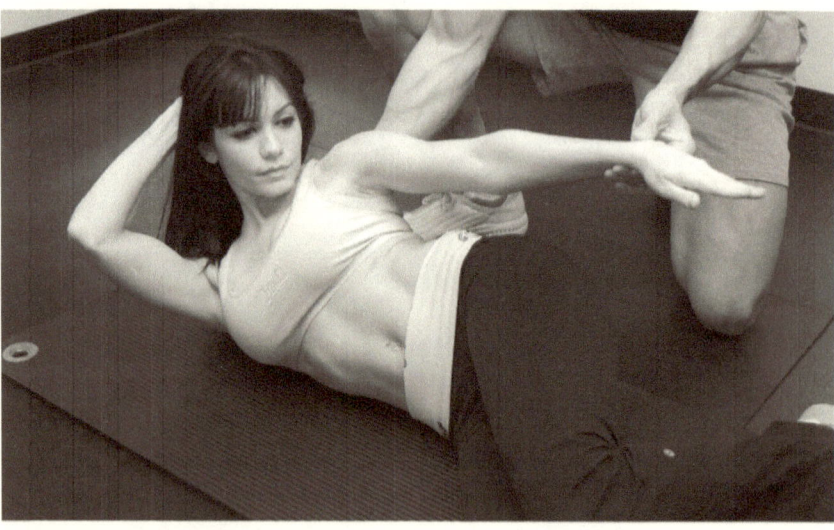

Freestanding Leg Raises with Knees Straight

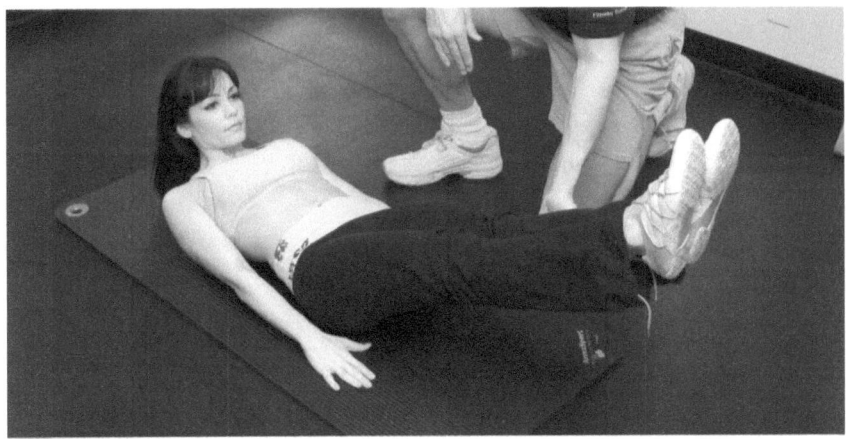

- Plant your arms firmly on the pads at the side for support.
- Place the small of your back on the lumbar support.
- Lift your legs horizontally, controlling each movement.
- Return to the starting position, controlling the movement.

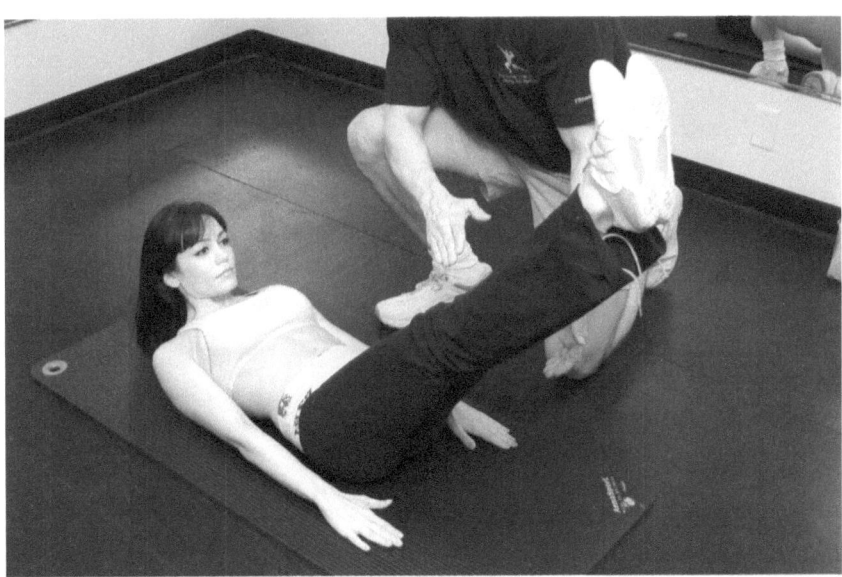

CHAPTER 8:
CORE TRAINING AND BALL EXERCISES

If you don't have access to a gym—or if you'd simply prefer to train in the privacy of your own home—you can invest in affordable training tools, such as an exercise/stability ball or training tubes and bands.

I'm a hardcore bodybuilder, and I'm also considered "old school." That means I train strictly with heavy weights and dumbbells. However, I became more open to the "new school" as I familiarized myself with new equipment, machines, and apparatuses. I also explored newer exercises and training methods.

When I started my personal training business in 2000, a fellow trainer introduced me to the exercise ball and other workout equipment. I also expanded my exercise knowledge by observing other trainers in the gym and noting what worked for their clients. I admit I was skeptical at first. The ball exercises looked easy, but once I started doing them myself, I found them challenging. I felt my muscles were being worked just as much as they were with free weights.

Working on the ball forces you to use precise technique. Your core must remain tight at all times, and you must maintain proper breathing.

Following are a variety of ball exercises that can give you a quality workout at the gym or at home. Here are some tips to remember when working with the exercise/stability ball:

- Keep your core and back tight when you're seated on the ball.
- Keep feet planted apart on the floor for stability and balance.
- Use lighter weights than usual.
- Do not use the same type of weight that you would if you were working on a bench or chair.
- Use a ball that's appropriate for your size.

First, here are basic floor exercises for effective core training, strength, and balance that can be done using an exercise/stability ball:

CORE TRAINING USING THE EXERCISE/STABILITY BALL

STABILITY BALL CURL

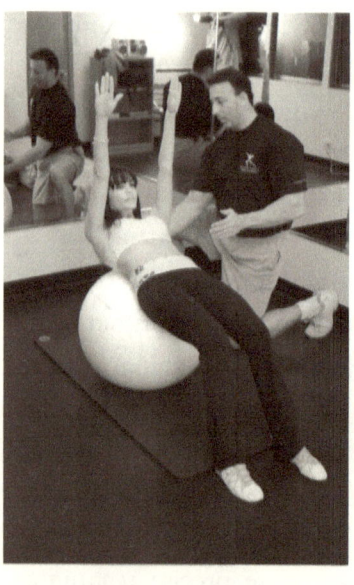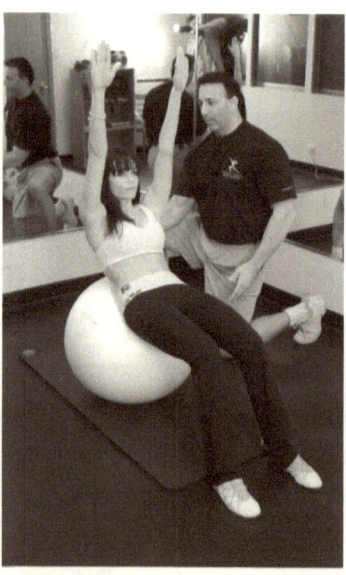

- Lie on the ball with both hands together and pointing upward.
- Contract your abdominal muscles.
- Curl your head and shoulders upward, keeping your hands moving directly upward.

CRUNCHES USING THE BALL TO SUPPORT FEET

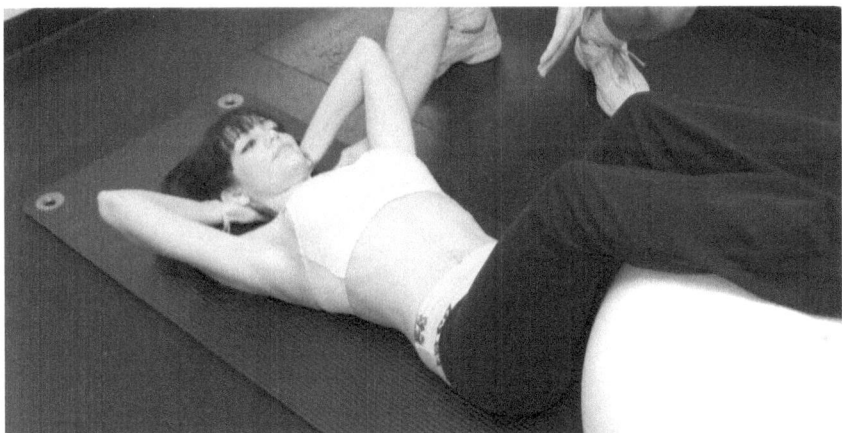

- Place your feet on the ball with your knees and hips bent at 90 degrees.
- Position your fingertips behind your head for support (but no yanking on your head!).
- Keep your shoulder blades off the ground.
- Contract your abdominal muscles and curl upward.

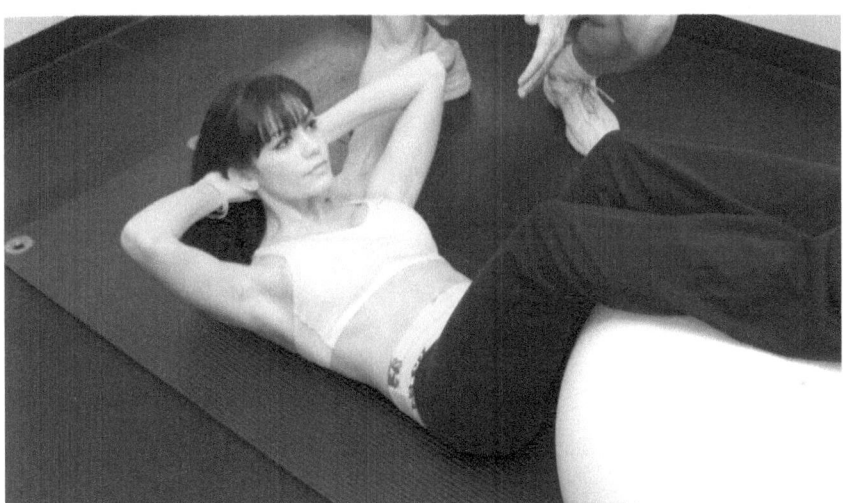

LEG RAISES WITH THE STABILITY BALL

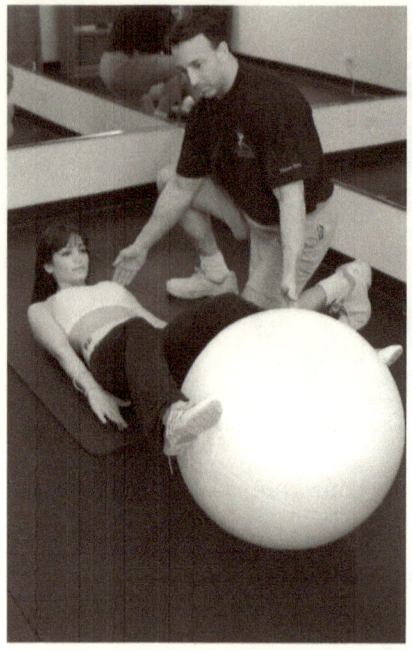 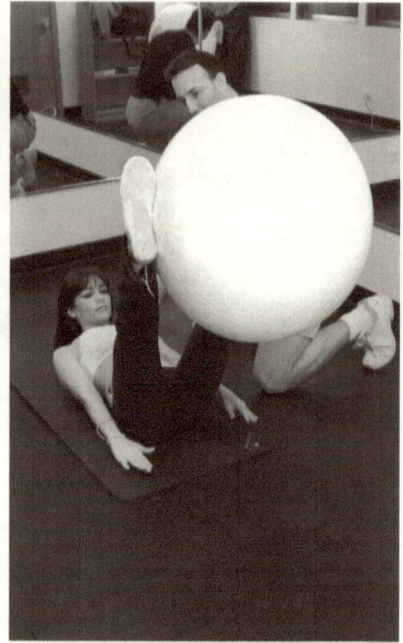

- Lie on your back and place the ball between your feet.
- Push your feet together to squeeze the ball.
- Keeping your hands to your sides, raise
  the ball to a 45-degree angle.

HIP-FLEXED ABDOMINAL CURL AND REACH

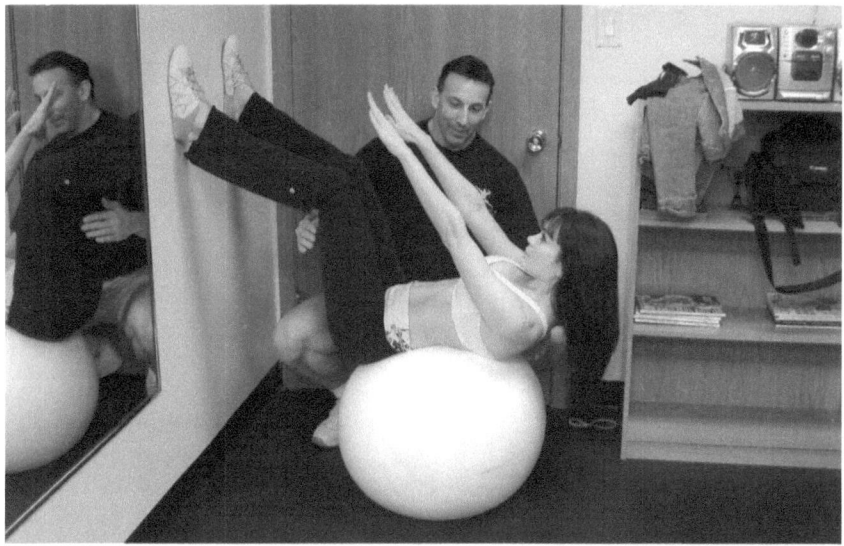

- Lie with your back flat on the ball.
- Elevate your feet on a wall.
- Contract your abdominals and reach upward with your hands, stretching as far as you can.

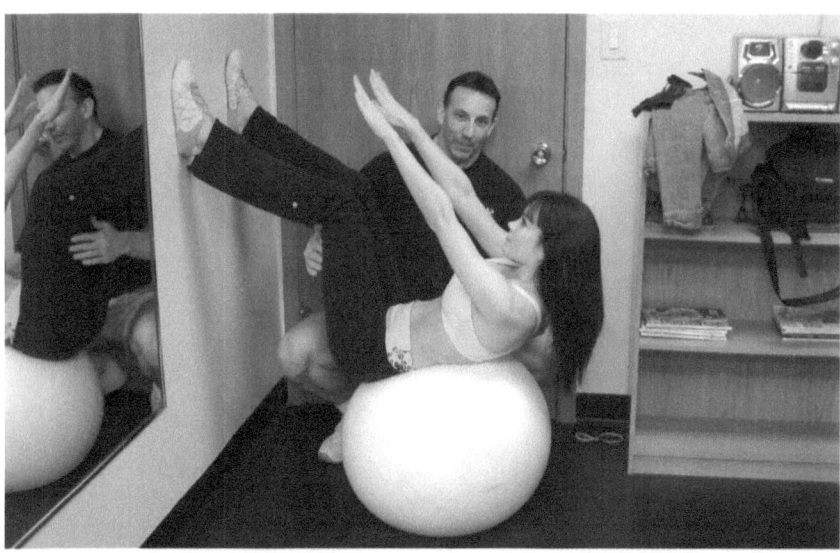

OBLIQUE LIFT

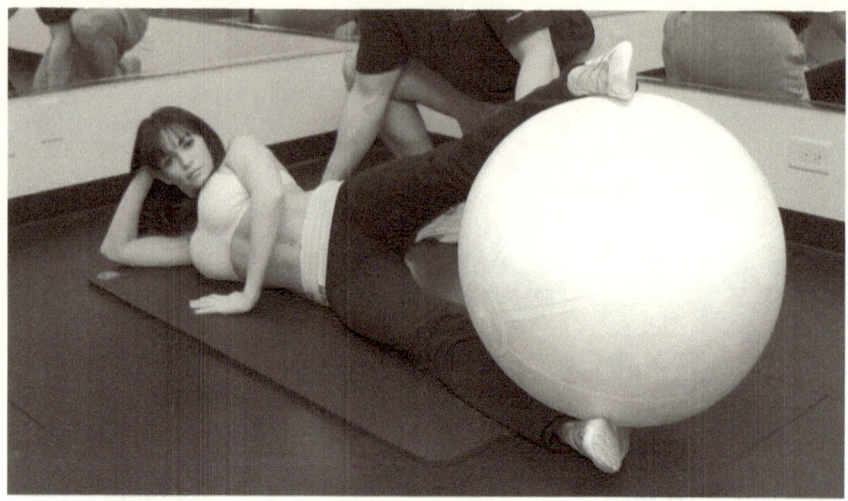

- Lie on your side with your head, shoulders, hips, and feet aligned.
- Place the ball between your feet.
- Contract your obliques to draw the ball upward toward your torso.

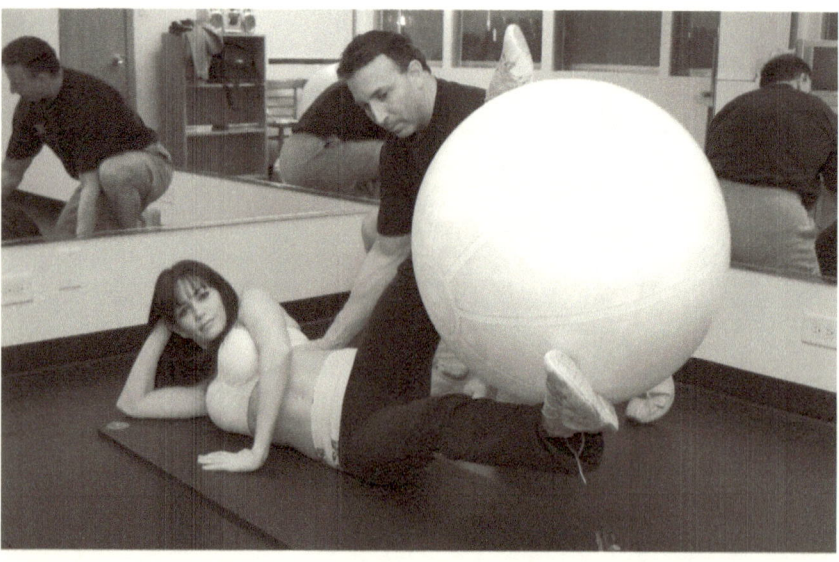

ROTATING THE TRUNK

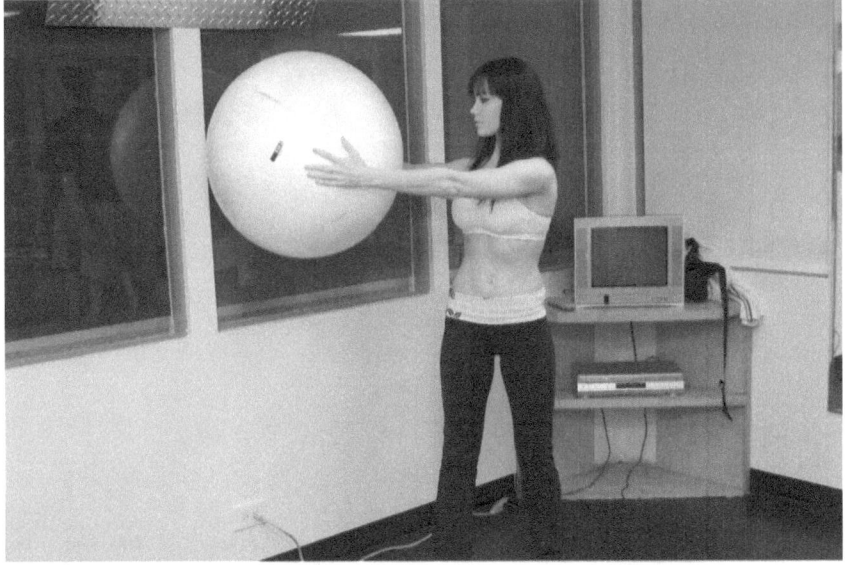

- Place your feet shoulder-width apart.
- Hold the ball with both hands, keeping your arms straight.
- Twist to one side and then the other, turning as far as possible.

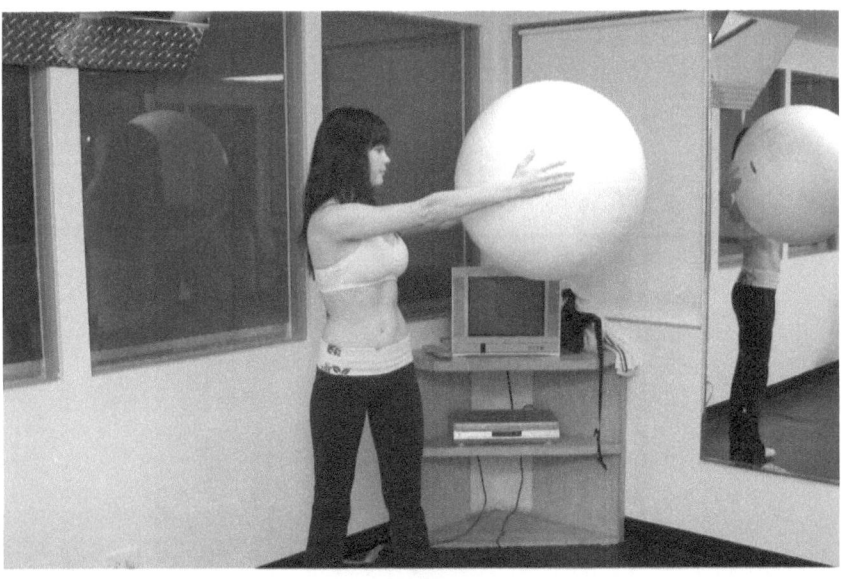

BALL EXERCISES FOR CHEST, SHOULDERS, BACK, BICEPS, AND TRICEPS

CHEST

Dumbbells Press

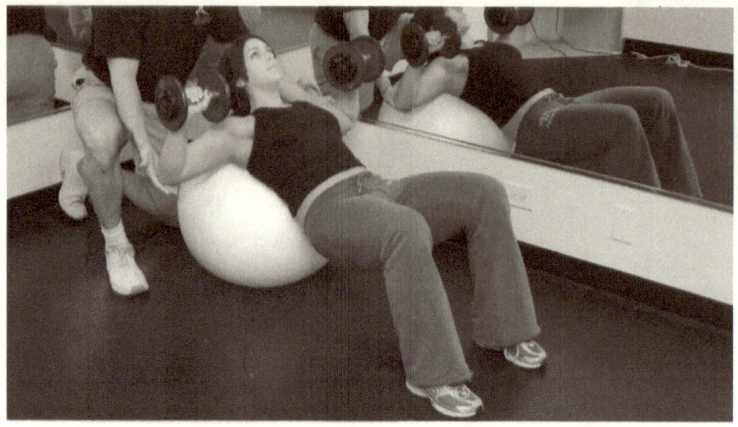

- Place your shoulders on the top center of the ball.
- Abdominals should be contracted, and head and spine should be lined up.
- Keep your hips up and your feet spread for solid balance.
- Drop your elbows and press, squeezing your chest muscles.

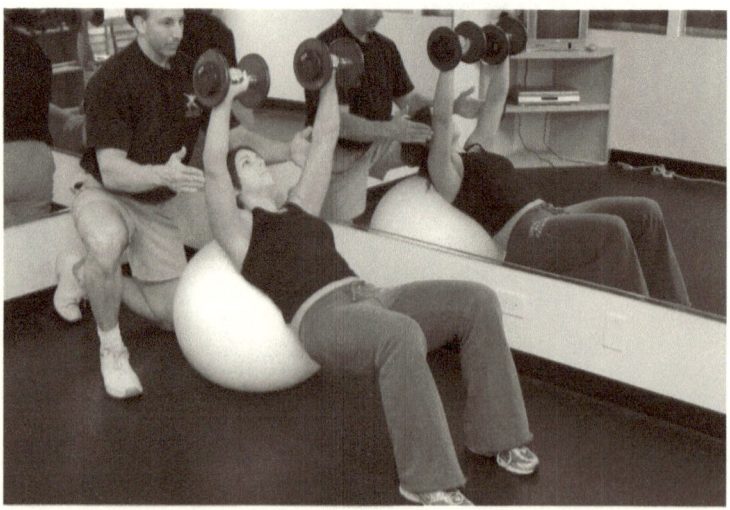

Incline Dumbbell Press

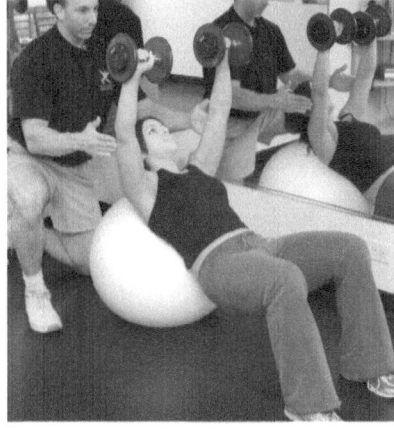
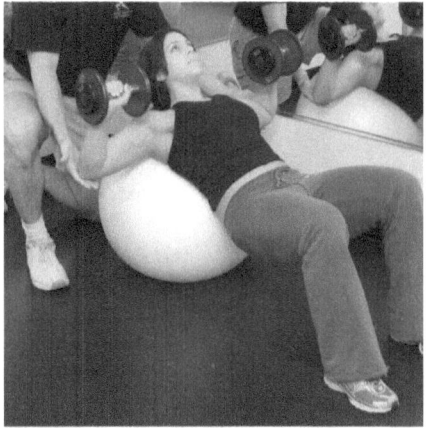

- Place your shoulders on the top center of the ball.
- Abdominals should be contracted.
- Lower your hips to a fist length above the ground so that your head, spine, and torso are on an incline.
- Drop your elbows and press, squeezing your upper chest muscles.

Push-Ups Using the Exercise Ball

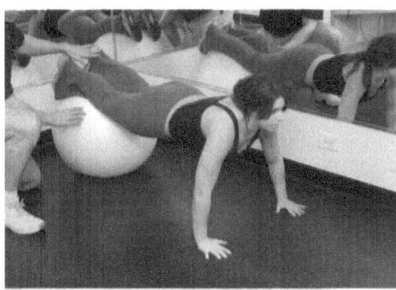
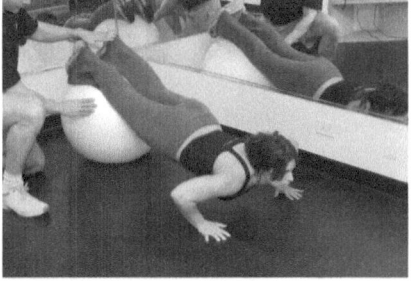

- Position your feet on top of the ball.
- Keep your back and your knees straight.
- Lower your chest to a fist length above the ground, then push up, straightening your elbows.

SHOULDERS

Shoulder Press

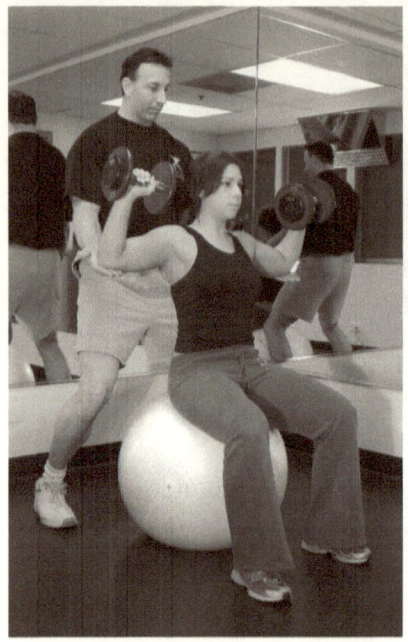 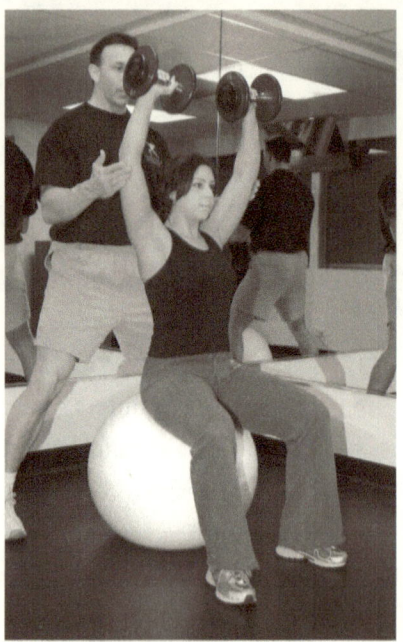

- Bring dumbbells down to your shoulders, then push your arms straight toward the ceiling.

Lateral Raises

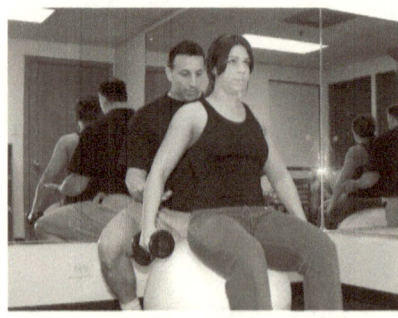 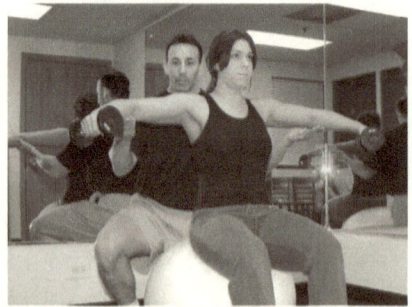

- With your arms slightly bent, raise arms to the side.
- Control both the upward and downward movements.

Rear Delts

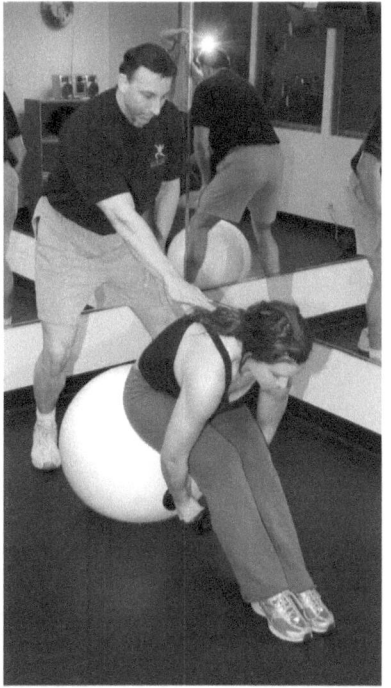 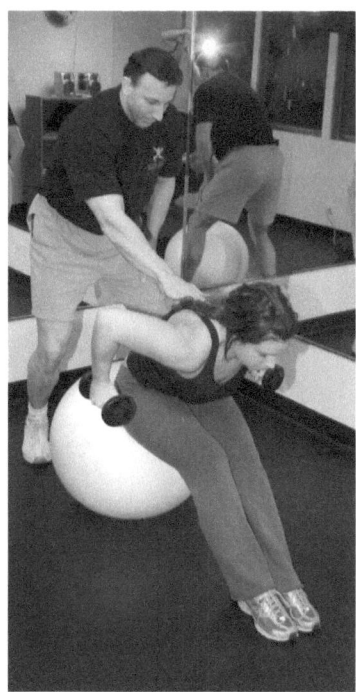

- Sit on the exercise ball.
- Straighten your legs out in front of you as far as you can.
- Hunch your body over, bringing your chest down toward your knees.
- Grab the dumbbells under your legs.
- Bring your arms straight back, leading with your elbows bent.

BICEPS

Alternating Dumbbell Curls

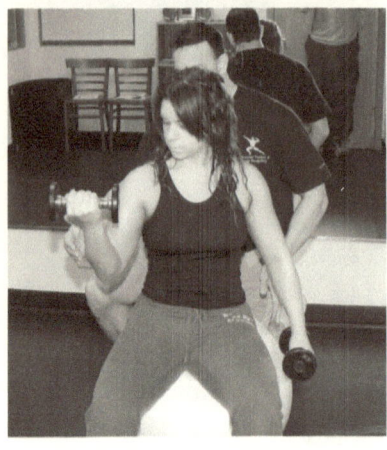 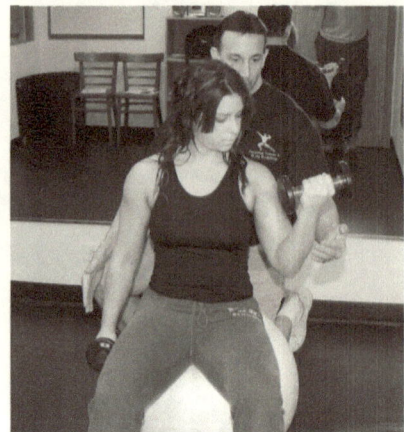

- Begin with your arms hanging down at the side of the ball.
- Curl one arm at a time, twisting your hand outward when the dumbbell reaches the leg.

One-Arm Dumbbell Curls

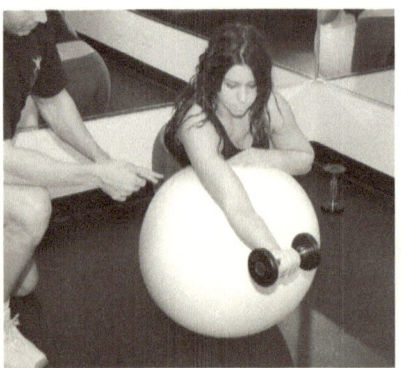 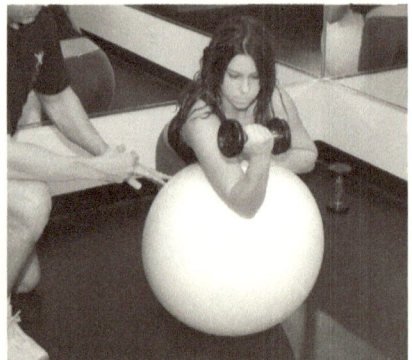

- Center your arm on the ball.
- Extend your arm downward and curl, squeezing the bicep.

Hammer Curls

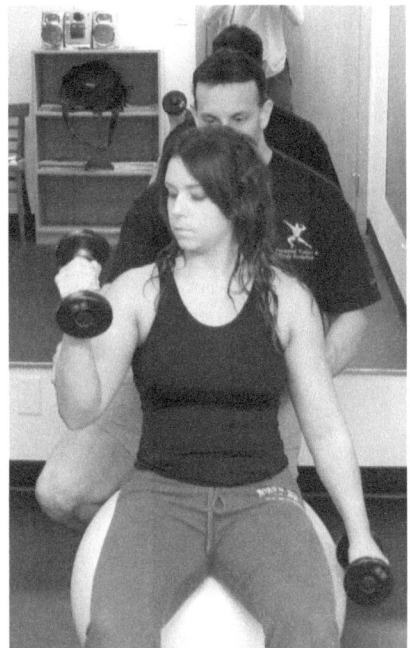 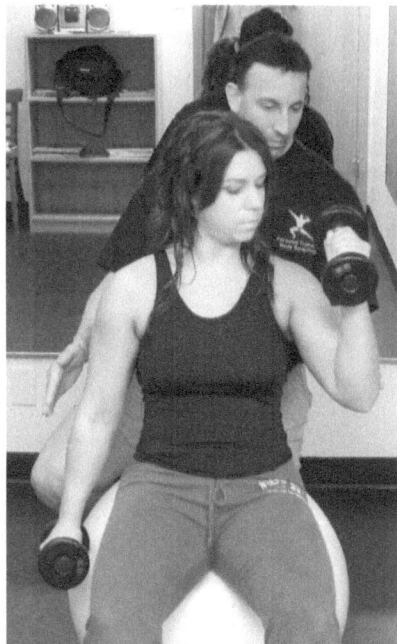

- Hold dumbbells as if you're holding a hammer.
- Bring your arms all the way up to the shoulder.

Triceps

Single-Arm Overhead Extension

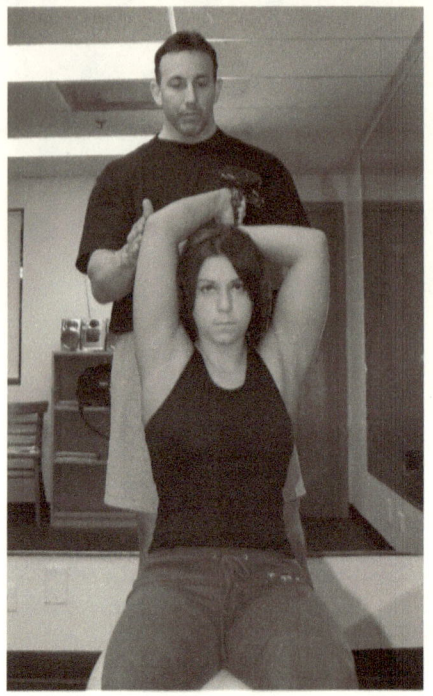 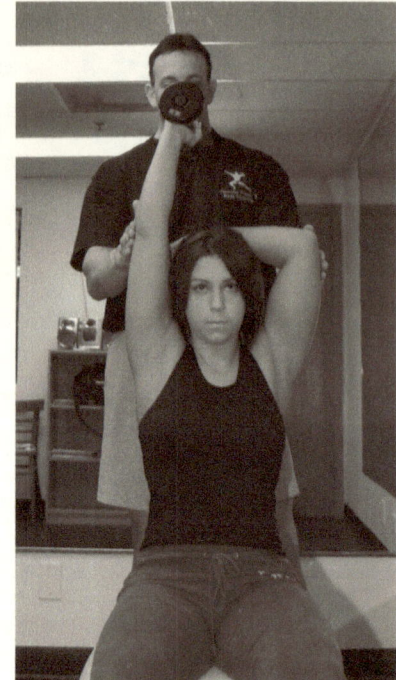

- Sit on the ball and bring one arm straight up so it's next to the ear on that side of the body.
- Bring the opposite arm up overhead and bend it at a 90-degree angle. Place that hand at the elbow of the straight arm.
- Lower the weight directly behind your head, then extend upward.

Tricep Kickbacks

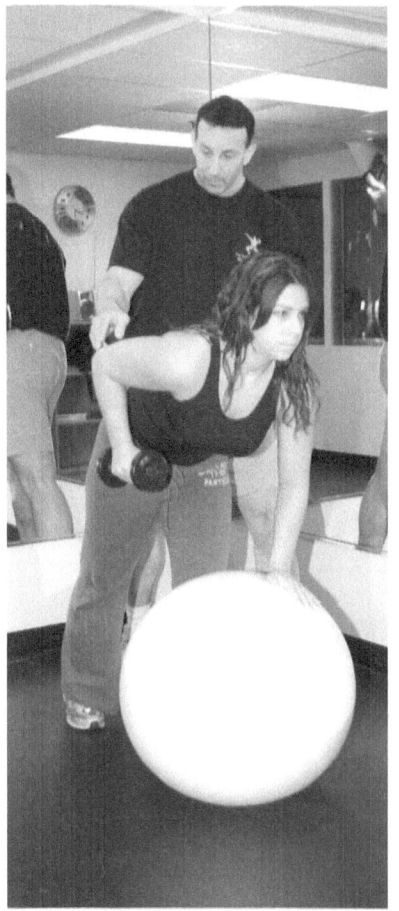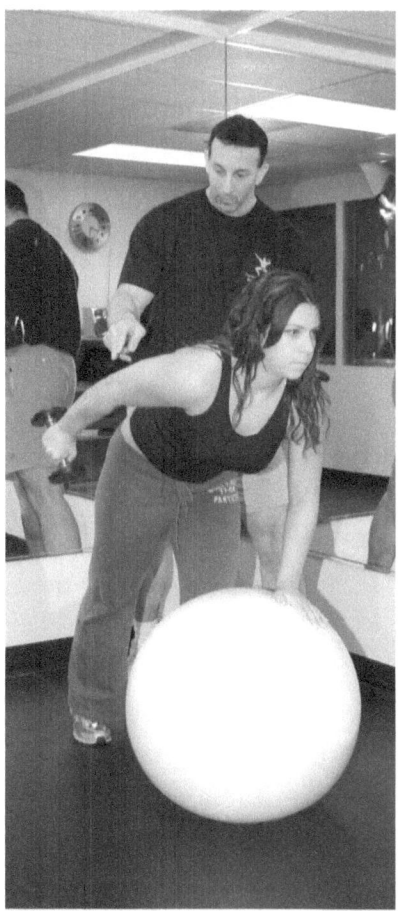

- Place one hand on the front of the ball.
- Place the knee on the same side of the body on the back of the ball.
- Keep your back straight.
- Bend your elbow 90 degrees to the side of the body.
- Extend your arm straight back, squeezing the tricep.
- Lower to the starting position.

BACK

One-Arm, Bent-Over Dumbbell Rows

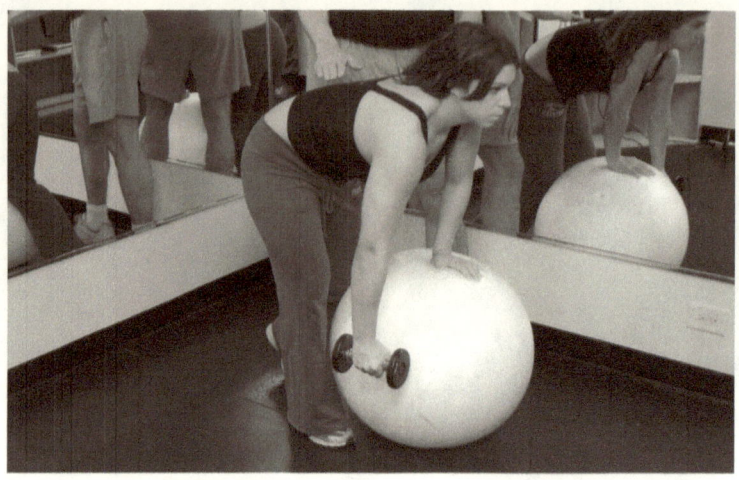

- Position one hand on the ball.
- Keep your feet shoulder-width apart, with one leg front and one leg back for balance.
- Place your front leg close to ball and to the hand that is supporting the body on the ball.
- Dip your other arm toward the floor.
- Pull your arm up, leading with the elbow and keeping your back straight.

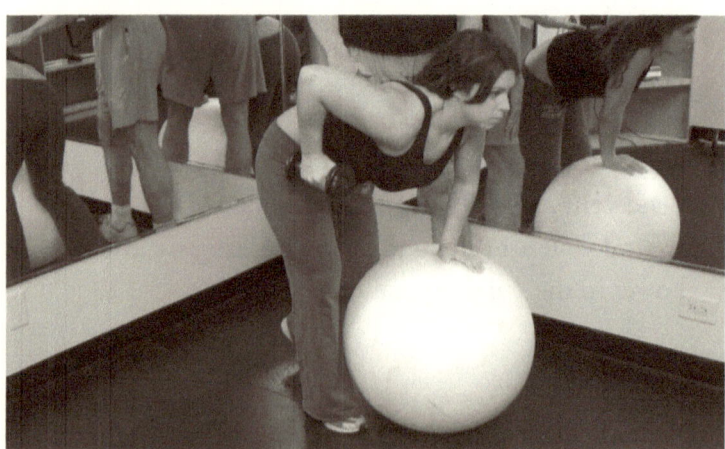

BACK

Alternating Arm and Leg Raise in Prone Position

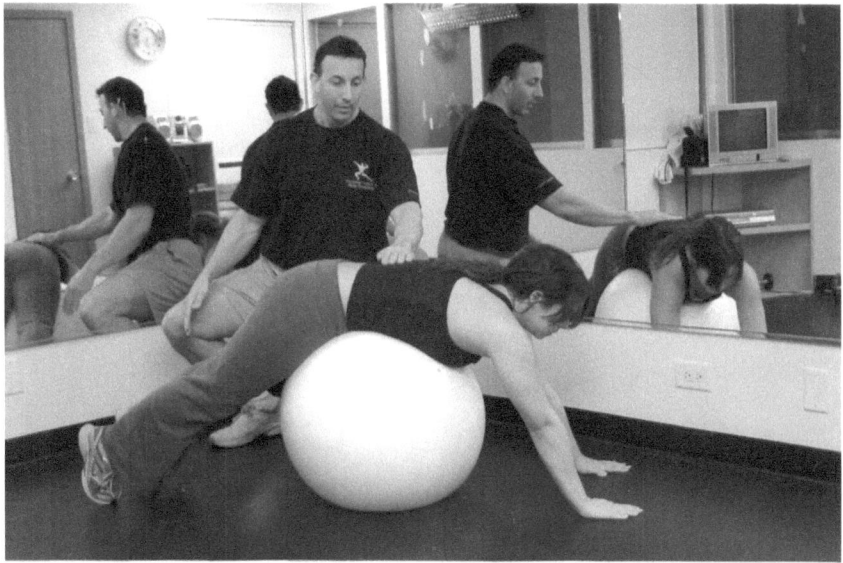

- Lie face down with your abs on the ball.
- Keep alternate hand and foot on the floor.
- Raise the opposite arm and leg simultaneously (i.e., lift your right arm and your left leg).

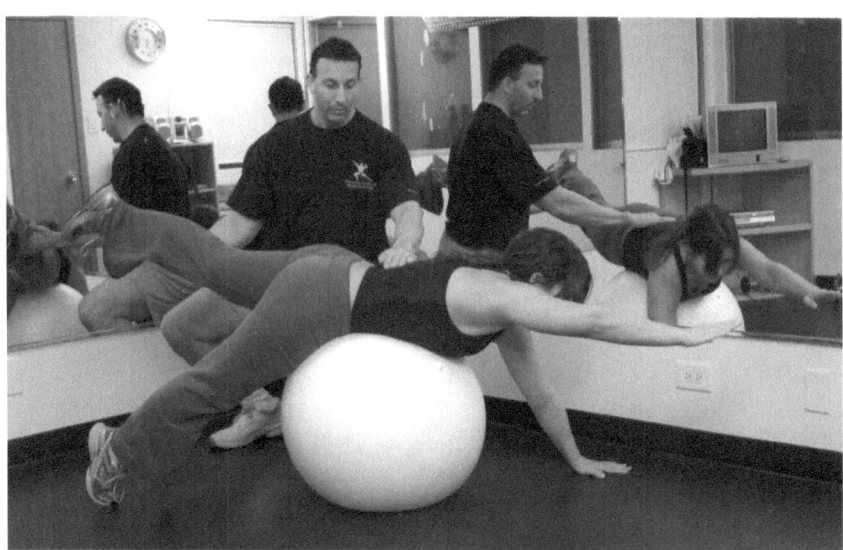

LEGS

Ball Squat Against the Wall

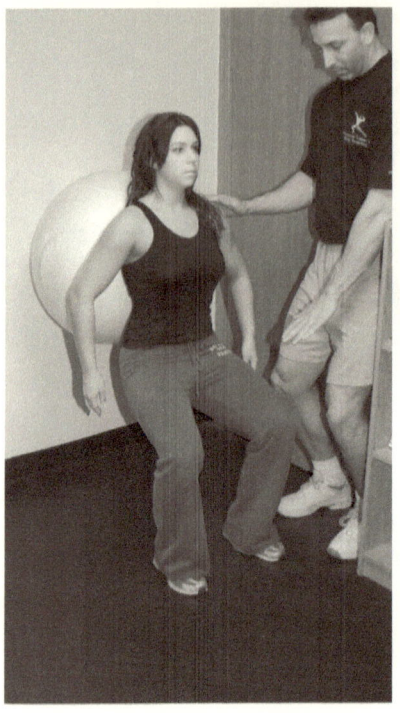 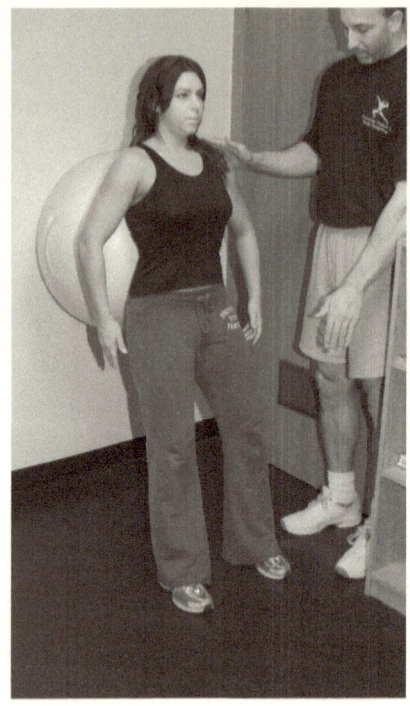

- Position the ball between the wall and your lower back while standing.
- Keeping your back straight, descend toward the floor with your arms out.
- Lower your body until your knees are bent 90 degrees.

Lunges

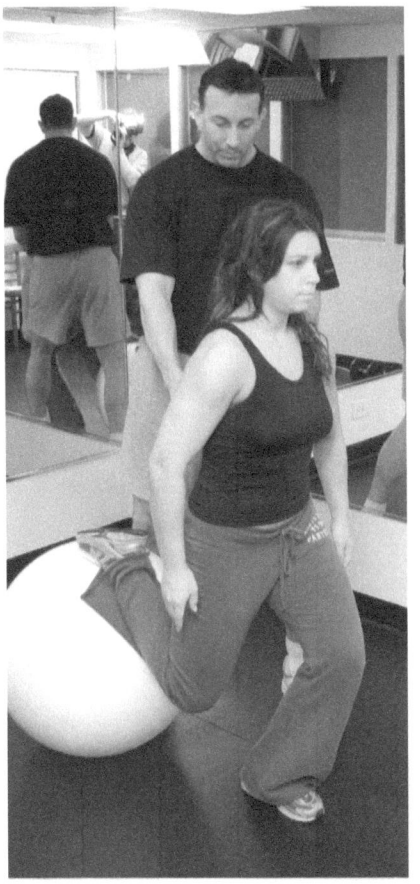 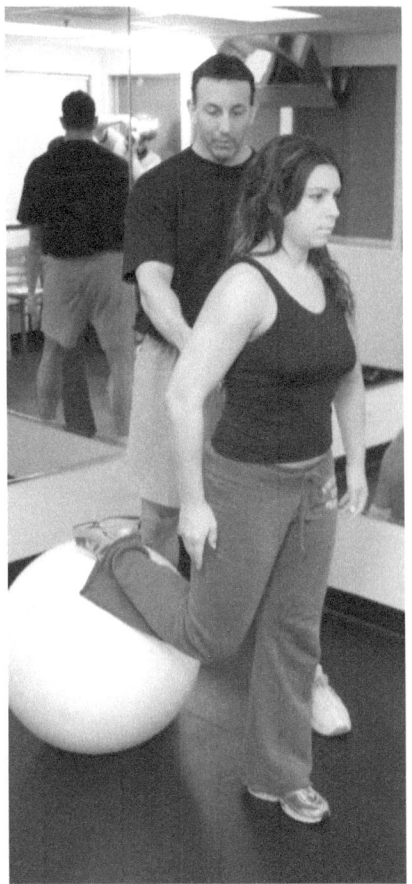

- Place one leg on the ball with the knee
  bent to a 90-degree angle.
- Keep legs shoulder-width apart.
- Bend your other knee, going as low as possible.
- Don't let your knee go forward over your foot.

Abductor Lift

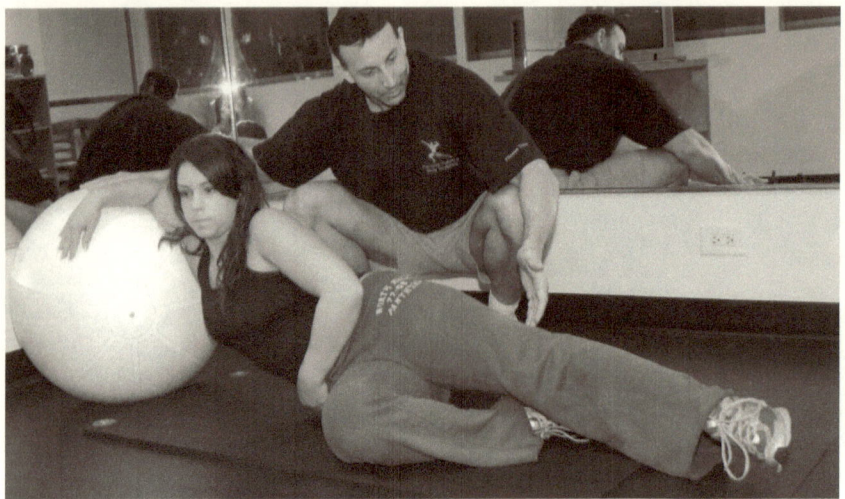

- Lean against the ball. Maintain your balance.
- Bend the knee closest to the ball 90 degrees.
- Straighten your other leg and lift it straight upward.
- Lower your leg slowly without hitting the ground.
- Repeat the same movement with the opposite leg.

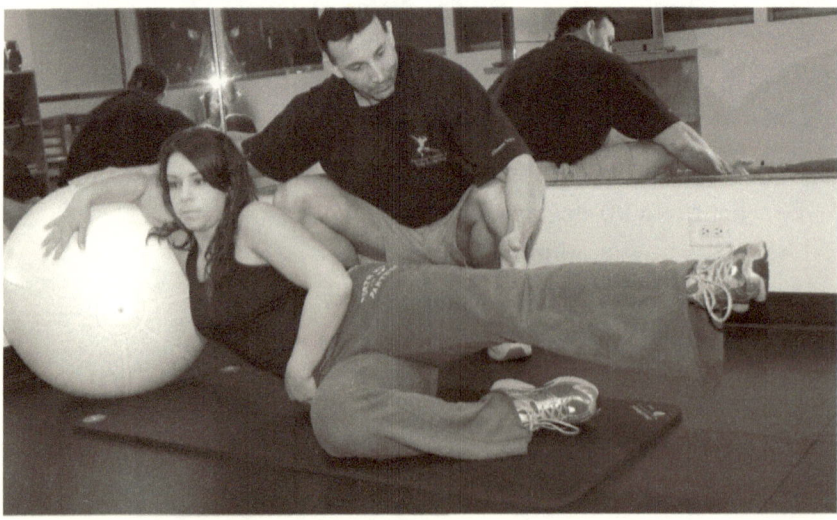

Adductor Squeeze

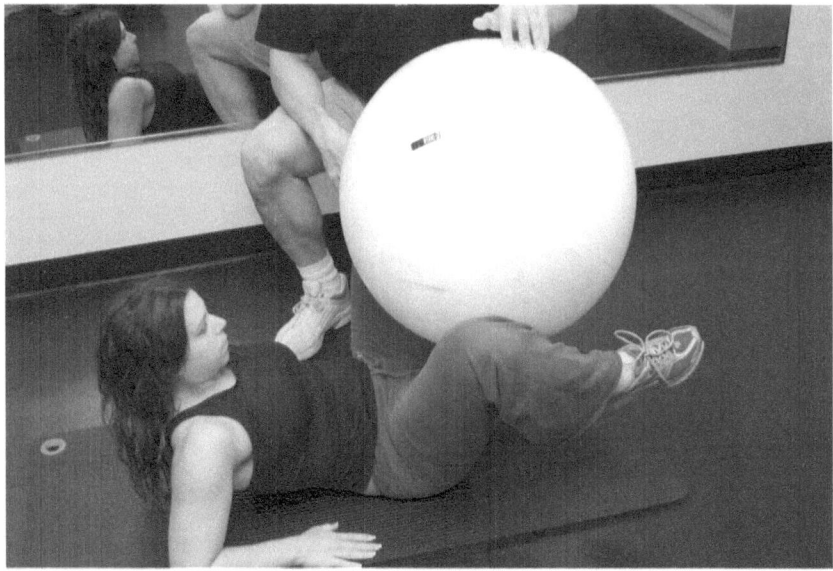

- Lie on your back and place ball between your knees.
- Squeeze the ball as tightly as possible.
- Keep your abdominals contracted.

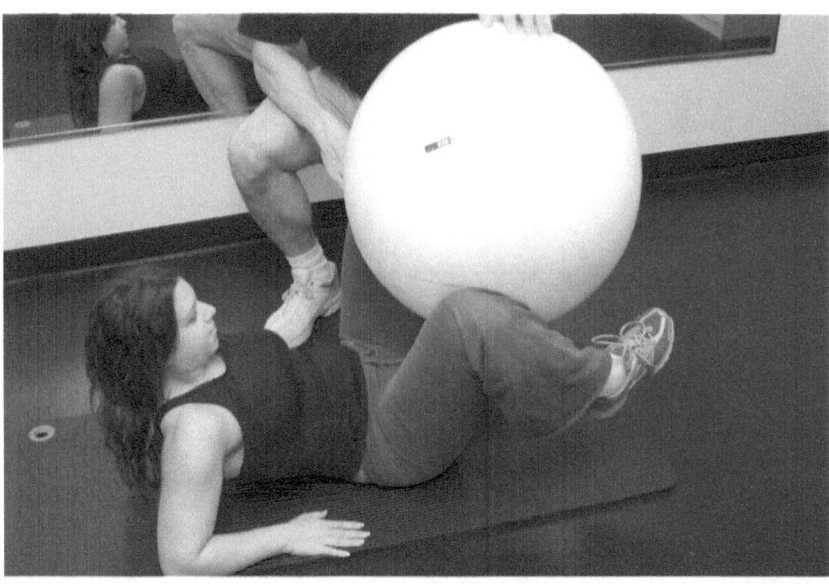

Ball Bridge Hip Extension

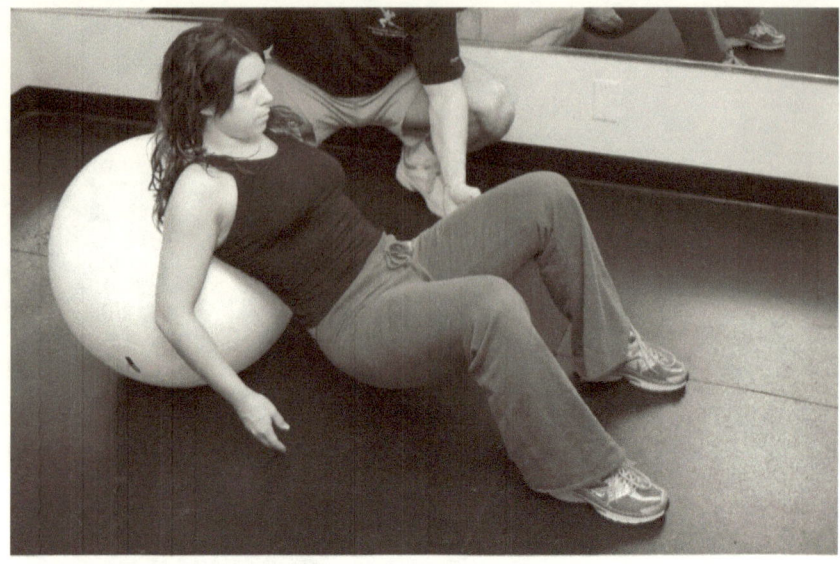

- Position your upper back on the ball.
- Keep your feet flat and your toes pointed straight ahead.
- Tighten your abs and keep your back straight.
- Lower your glutes without touching the floor.
- Squeeze the glutes, then return to the starting position.

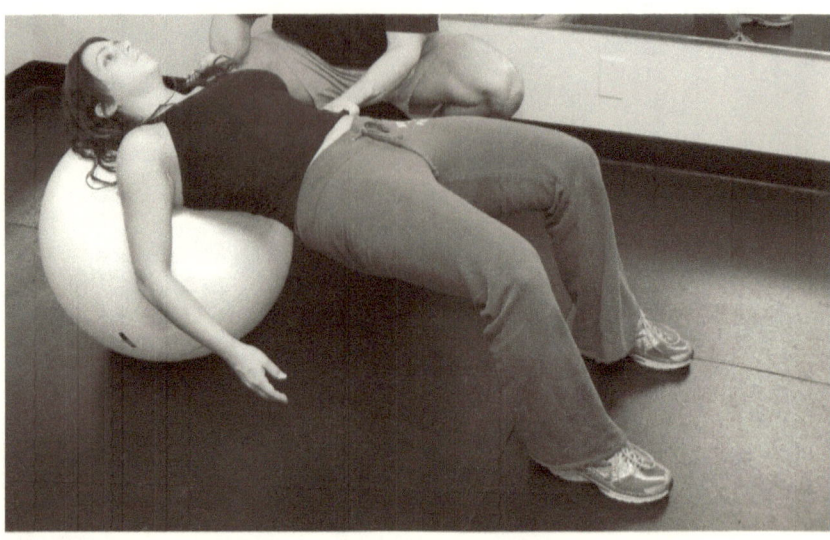

CHAPTER 9:
CONTINUING THE JOURNEY AND MOVING FORWARD

As a fitness professional, I continue to research and learn new techniques. I get new ideas from fellow fitness experts and through interaction with gym staff and members. I even discover new exercise techniques through trial and error.

My fitness journey was not easy, nor will it ever be easy. But my setbacks and trials stirred up my desire to show people that a real, average person like me can persevere and achieve a good physique the "old-fashioned way." I'm grateful that I've been at "both ends of the spectrum" so that I can encourage people and show others that good health and fitness are possible.

I am often asked, "What will happen to your muscle if you stop training?" Unused muscle simply atrophies; it does not turn into fat. People become fat when they stop exercising because they don't reduce their caloric intake to match their lower activity level. But I'm glad people ask that question. My standard answer is: "The words 'stop training' don't exist in my vocabulary."

I've been training for more than half of my life, and I love it! I would never think about stopping. I don't care how busy my life is—I still get myself to the gym or do some aerobic activity. I plan to keep my physique in the best shape possible, no matter what my age. It is not wise to stop training when you get older, or to come up with excuses. Each year, there will be more obstacles to overcome. The older the body gets, the greater the risk of muscle atrophy. That's why I will always be committed to setting goals. I encourage everyone to keep striving to reach the next level—not only in fitness, but in all areas of life. I'm very blessed to have encountered special people who are in their 80s and who are still setting goals and continuing to live life with passion.

I did a lot of thinking when I was confined to a hospital bed in 1999 after my martial arts injury. I felt that it was time to transition from martial arts into bodybuilding, since I had accomplished all the martial arts goals that I had set. My new fitness goals were to gain muscle mass and compete in a bodybuilding contest. I have competed in ten competitions since writing this book; I will say that *I am not done yet*!

I have many more goals that I would like to attain in all areas of my life. Being fit will help me achieve those goals and live life to the fullest. There is a plaque hanging in my kitchen that I look at every morning when I'm eating my egg whites and oatmeal. On it is a quote from Abraham Lincoln: "It is not the years in your life, but the life in your years." By being healthy and fit, *you* can have a fulfilling life journey, too.

Remember, there are no quick fixes. It is a journey. It takes sacrifice, but the rewards and benefits will be well worth the time and money you invest. Stop making excuses! Motivate yourself to make the changes you need to make. Apply the principles and techniques in this book so that you, too, can be "living proof."

Now get out there and take that journey!

www.ingramcontent.com/pod-product-compliance
Lightning Source LLC
Chambersburg PA
CBHW020240290526
45784CB00003B/1049